MW01285593

"I love Logan's story. I love h
with people. Few of us have
relate, in one way or another. Logan inspires, period."

Brant Hansen — Christian Radio personality who hosts his
own nationally broadcasted show, and author of the book,
"Unoffendable."

"Logan, you ARE "The Difference Maker" in the lives of others
that my father (Zig Ziglar) spent his life encouraging people to
become. You perfectly exemplify the attitude that Dad wanted
his readers to embrace."

Julie Ziglar Norman — Author and Daughter of renowned inspirational and motivational speaker, Zig Ziglar. He authored many
books, and included Logan Shannon in his book, "Embrace the
Struggle".

"Logan's book is essential for all of us to read. It changed my life
perspective every day I turned a page. I even implemented the
daily practice of praying aloud because of what Logan wrote.
Eternally grateful for the gift Logan has given us."

Eric Anthony Ceislewicz — Producer for the EntreLeadership Podcast

"Logan, *that's* the secret to moving on with life. The weaker we
are, the harder we must lean on Jesus; and the harder we lean
on Him, the stronger we discover Him to be."

Joni Eareckson Tada — Founder and CEO of Joni and Friends
International Disability Center, is an international advocate for
people with disabilities. Joni has written over 50 books and has
received the Gold Medallion Lifetime Achievement Award from
the Evangelical Christian Publishers Association.

THE LOGAN LETTERS

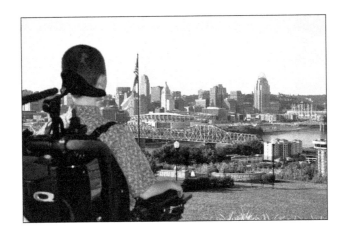

LOGAN SHANNON
with LEE H. KRESSER

THE LOGAN LETTERS

Every Experience Has Endless Impact

LOGAN SHANNON
with LEE H. KRESSER

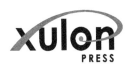

*This book is gratefully dedicated to my
Mom and Dad, Tyra and Michael Shannon,
my sister, Sydney;
and my brothers, Devon and Corey
for all their support, love, understanding and patience
as I travel this road through life.
You all have shared what it's like to know Christ,
and to live in Christ.*

*And thank You, Lord.
You brought me into this world to make a difference,
and I didn't quite expect it to be this way.......
Thank You!*

*And thank you to my dear friends who helped me through the
years and those who wrote letters for this book.*

"Trust in the Lord with all your heart and lean not on your
own understanding. In all your ways acknowledge Him,
and He shall direct your paths."
Proverbs 3:5-6

This book contains a **great video play feature** hidden in both picture sections after each intermission and in chapter 21 on pages 242 and 247.

Wikitude allows a reader to position a smart phone over designated pages, take the "picture" of the page while holding it, and watch a prepared video directly from that page. Follow these instructions:

Step 1 – Download free Wikitude app

Step 2 – Enter search code for the page you want to view
(A drop-down selection may appear prior to entering the complete search code. Pick one or complete the entry and only one selection for that search code will remain)

Step 3 – Click on the file name after entering the search code

Step 4 – Hold the smart phone over the designated page and click to watch Logan's video! Do not move away from the page.

Video #1 slide show from the first picture section after first intermission (see note on that page)
Enter code: LogLetterEY (for Early Years) – 1st int)

Video #2 slide show from the second picture section after the second intermission (see note on that page)
Enter code: LogLetterLY (for Later Years) – 2nd int)

Video #3 Watch video from Logan's 2013 high school commencement speech as one of the co-valedictorians (Chapter 22)
Enter code: LogLetterHSG (for High School Graduation)

Video #4 Watch video from Logan's inspirational message to a church youth group (Chapter 22) Enter code: LogLetterYM (for Youth Message)

E-books will be equipped with a hyperlink to watch each video.

Table of Contents

An Opening Word

Dear Reader,

That's you. Yes, you! After all, you are reading this, right?! As you begin turning these pages, here's what you need to know: This book is just as much about your story as it is my story! In fact, it isn't much about me at all; my story is meant to be a tool for you to use to overcome your own hardships and develop a new understanding of what your purpose in this life is.

Look at my story as a blueprint of sorts to find real meaning in the world around you and to use your life, namely your weaknesses and subsequent perseverance, as a source of inspiration and courage to the ones you come in contact with every day. I realize this may not be the case with all, but my hope is that one of your main takeaways to achieve these things, is your need for Jesus Christ as your Savior and to allow him to have full reign in your life. That's the core of the message, and that I won't shy away from!

In order to stick with this blueprint idea, my friend Lee, is going to serve as your guide to looking into my life throughout the entirety of the book. What better way to help you overcome and inspire in response to my experiences than to be led by another who already claims that he has done so simply by being a witness to my everyday life? For the most part, the perspective you'll be hearing is Lee's, an outsider looking in if you will. And in your case isn't that exactly what position you're in as well?

Don't worry though, you will be hearing plenty of my voice 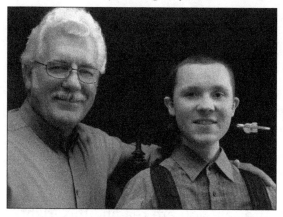 along the way in the form of, you guessed it... letters! You'll also be coming across more letters from my family, friends, and other acquaintances, more outsiders looking in that you can relate to. May this whet your appetite to peer into my life in order for you to become the hero of your story that we have all been created to be as a means to point the world to the one true Hero!

Your Friend,
Logan

Foreword by Julie Ziglar Norman

(Daughter of Zig Ziglar)

Dear Logan,

I will always cherish the day Mom, Dad and I finally got to meet you and the rest of your beautiful family in person. We felt like we had known all of you for years. When you rolled into the green room, with the rest of the crew in tow, at the "Get Motivated Seminar" where Dad and I were speaking in Cincinnati, Ohio; the bond of friendship and kinship was powerfully present. That is how it is when people share their personal struggles and the faith that sustains them.

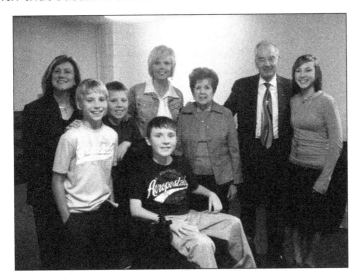

You were thirteen-years-old when my father, motivational speaker and author, Zig Ziglar fell down the stairs in his home and had a brain injury that devastated his short term memory. Living with the challenges of his brain injury led Dad to write *Embrace the Struggle: Living Life on Life's Terms*, a book of encouragement and inspiration for folks who were struggling to accept life circumstances they could not change or wish away. Dad asked me to help him write the book and I was seeking stories for a chapter about individuals who were positively living with disabilities that they were born with when my brother told me he knew the perfect person to write about.

Tom Ziglar (Zig's son) said that your father had told your story

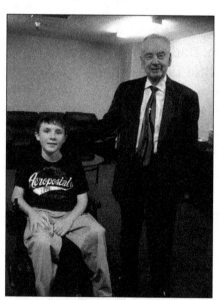

and how God had sustained you and your family at our Ziglar Inc., Monday morning devotional. I called your father and asked if he and your mom would be willing to share your family's journey in Dad's book. The friendship and shared prayers of our families has remained constant ever since. Your mom has sent me a Christmas card and a new family picture every year since 2008. I hung that first picture on my desk as a daily reminder to pray for you and your family.

I taped each new picture to the bottom of the previous year until it got so long I had to move all the pictures to the wall beside my desk. I love seeing how you, Sydney, Devon and Corey have grown and matured through the years and I look forward to opening your family Christmas card every year.

I have been deeply blessed to pray for all of you and I have treasured the close friendship that developed between me and your mom. She has proudly shared your milestones with me and I wept with pride as I watched your Valedictorian speech. I felt the joy of your parents as I know they marveled at the depth of your character, the strength of your purpose and the passion with which you live your life. I was proud to see how mature you are, the true leader of others you have become and to be included in the celebration of your achievement.

Logan, you ARE "The Difference Maker" in the lives of others that my father spent his life encouraging people to become. You perfectly exemplify the attitude that Dad wanted his readers to embrace.

Your can-do, will-do, and done-deal lifestyle totally destroys most people's excuses for not doing more with the life they've been given. You have inspired me, the faith of your family has inspired me and I know God is using all of you mightily to inspire and encourage others.

God bless you and always remember: ***Because He lives... we can face tomorrow***.

> Joshua 1:9 – "Have I not commanded you? Be strong and of good courage; do not be afraid, nor be dismayed, for the LORD your God *is* with you wherever you go."

In His bountiful love,
Julie Ziglar Norman

Introduction

Who is Logan Shannon? Why would his life be special? Why would someone like a renowned speaker named Zig Ziglar find Logan's life and those of his family worth writing about in a book?

The reason Logan's story needed to be told is because he has impacted so many people in his twenty two year life. His boundless energy in his very early years with his sister and brothers began to change as he showed signs of a disease that would eventually put him in a wheelchair. You'll see pictures of his leg casts and leg braces as the disease gradually took its toll. You'll sense the frustrations of coping with the tightening grip of immobility and the realization that he would have to abandon many of life's activities.

At the same time, you will also see how his faith in God and complete trust in Jesus Christ has placed him in a position of incredible influence and credibility. He has been pushed to the brink, and held on. His family has been hit from many angles because of their wrestling with health issues, agencies, inconveniences, altered dreams, frustration, exhaustion and fatigue, and financial tsunami's. And yet the entire family understands that Logan *is* family. There is no other alternative. He is intertwined in the arguments, celebrations, travels, disciplines, passions, and rewards of his family. And their faith has bonded them together with a deeply spiritual stitching where they can laugh together or cry together as they travel down this unique road.

This book isn't about childish pranks like young brothers knowing where the green peas mysteriously went from the dinner plate, or who ate the chocolate. Logan's contribution is much more than that. He may be remembered **because** he's in a wheelchair, and **could** be remembered as such. But that's not important. He is to be remembered because of how he made other people *feel*. Logan is witty, complex, wise, insightful, educated, perceptive, and loving. He is dedicated to his friends and their friendships, he recognizes his place in this life, and he strongly believes that he will take whatever condition the Lord has him endure.

You'll read how he was there at a basketball game with a friend who has Cerebral Palsy, and cheered him on with encouragement. You'll read how many fellow students in school wondered why there was always a shortage of available seats at the cafeteria table where Logan was seated because there were so many kids who wanted to be around him. You'll read how fellow students wanted him to be the school mascot, and actually designed and built a Roman Chariot structure (complete with horses) for his wheelchair so he could race up and down the football game sidelines leading cheers on for his school team.

So, yeah, Logan Shannon *is* in a wheelchair. And so what! It

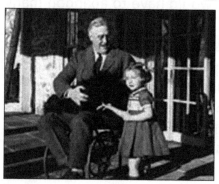

doesn't matter what the reason is, right? If he rolled up to you in a store, in a school, or in a sports venue, what would you do? If he was in line for something like you were, what would you say? Would you look and turn away? Would you stare, and try to figure out what the issue was? Or would you decide to greet him, and actually treat him like ANY other person? But I assure you, Logan Shannon is a person you would WANT to meet. And so is every other individual with a disability for that matter. That's the way it ought to be. That's the way it is, at least when we don't let our "normalcy" get in the way, that is. And besides, did you know that we happen to have had a president who required a wheelchair?

Franklin Delano Roosevelt was the president of the United States elected to four terms in the last century, who contracted polio at a young age. Because of arrangements with the media, he was always photographed or filmed so a wheelchair would

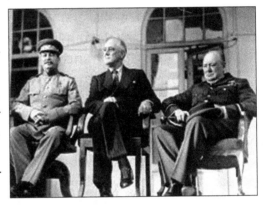

not be seen. Why not? Because some would come to incorrect conclusions due to the presence of a wheelchair. Back then, a wheelchair had implications of weakness. In fact, only a few photos even exist showing the president in a wheelchair.

Even during meetings with world leaders, President Roosevelt would be seen seated in a regular chair, much of the time with his legs crossed. When filmed standing, he would be propped up while speaking. Times have changed in many ways, but human nature hasn't. You couldn't talk to Roosevelt then and can't now.

But at the FDR memorial in Washington, DC, there's a bronze

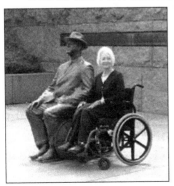

statue there with him cast actually IN a wheelchair. There were instructions for the memorial that it be designed so those with different disabilities could experience it. In fact, many visitors with some inabilities of some kind are photographed with that bronze figure of the president in his wheelchair for personal reasons.

There are so many people with disabilities, suffered through accidents, infirmities due to disease, war injuries, and conditions from birth that the person couldn't control. They have a story, and EVERYONE has value! When we see people or meet people, we size them up right away, don't we? We make decisions from what we see immediately. We make these judgments about people and situations based on partial data; and consequently, we can be way wrong sometimes. And many times, we've squandered wonderful opportunities to experience truly fascinating people, haven't we?

If a man has facial scars, will some ladies turn away before they find out he saved a family of six from a house fire?

If a woman's appearance isn't totally captivating, will many pass her up, scanning the horizon for another selection that meets a quality that will naturally disappear with time?

There are many "Logans" out there, waiting to be talked to, laughed with, joked with, or suffered alongside.

Here's a question: "What if we decide too quickly about a person, and we miss out on one of the most treasured people in our lives?" Or what if I re-phrase that question: "How many times have we made a decision about someone before we really knew what the person was really like?"

Every reader will be moved by this way of thinking, in some way. But how many will reflect back and remember a callous remark, a practical joke that bordered on cruel, or regret a missed chance that could have brought happiness and peace into their own lives? And how many will smile when they can recall the times they opened their hearts and asked a person INTO their lives that wasn't like themselves just ***because***.

And so it is with Logan Shannon. He is one of those rare characters who can be with such a variety of people and dissipate anxiety, who can encourage in ways that defy logic, who can adapt and be part of a joke, who can cry with you when you are grieving for some reason; and he can reach out to those who don't know him in a relaxed attitude of open invitation.

People **want** to be around this guy. I do! Strangers have been known to admire him, before they had even met him. Spend a little time with this book, and find out how these Logan Letters touch you. Who knows, there may be someone out there right now just like Logan waiting for you to approach them with respectful curiosity and authenticity. Are you ready to meet them?

If I **tell** you a story, you may remember it. If I **write** a story and give it to you, it will mean so much more. Why? Because I can choose to read it slowly. Or I can re-read it at my leisure to get a deeper meaning to its words. Or I can choose to put it down and resume the story at a later date. But if I tell you a story, you have to be totally engaged at that exact moment to listen to each chosen word, or you may get done before I am.....

Also if I tell a story about another person, and you don't know that other person; that unknown person's facial appearance and expressions will never be known. So throughout this book, you will not only read Logan's letters to others, you will read those other people's letters to Logan; complete with pictures through the years.

Logan wants to share his life with you, and share what impact he has made with others. So he offers these brief letters / testimonies as examples. Who knows, some readers may even use these as an example to reach out and express to someone else in their world who may need a thoughtful reminder of the importance of the relationship that's theirs.

As you "open" and read each of these letters, you'll also open a part of yourself that allows Logan to reach into your life and embrace you. Can his arms physically do that? Not necessarily.... Turn the pages, letting the stories roll into your mind, leading you into Logan's life, and you'll see....

Chapter 1

Letters, Important Messages from the Past

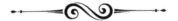

Everyone has a story. What's **your** story? Is it filled with heartache or adventure? Is it filled with poverty or wealth? Are you an only child who may have been orphaned, or one in a huge family where reunions can be total chaos? Remember, we **all** are part of someone else's story.

Now what if someone could open the hidden grandstand of cheering family and friends, and watch you secretly stand up for a bullied kid at school or an intimidated co-worker? What if we could pull back the curtains and watch how you reached out to a troubled soul and shared a heavy burden to lighten their load? What would they think when you chose to be honest when **no one** was looking? What if we saw in your actions that you really made a difference in other people's lives? I think many of us could. And many wish they had.

So, is your story filled with sadness and regret? Is it filled with happiness and fulfillment? Has it taken a dark turn with a diagnosis of cancer or some other disease? Or has your life gone from a tough, hopeless, battle-worn existence to one of peace and gratitude?

What would you do if someone could peel back the covering of your life? Would you feel embarrassed? Would you feel like you wasted a ton of time? Would you see yourself in a different light, and objectively try to do things better with the time you had left?

Here's the big question: How will we ever know if someone actually lived, <u>unless</u> there was evidence. Right? Take for example, George Washington. Has anyone currently living ever met him? Is he real? Of course! Why? There's evidence! There are pictures and documents that verify his existence and personal contributions to forming our country.

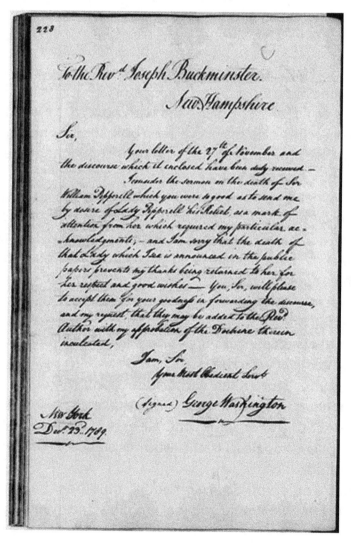

Was he perfect? No. He was the eldest of his nine siblings and born in 1732. His voice would never be recorded. Yet his words ring out into history as a military leader and key figure in the creation of the United States federal government.

George Washington was a statesman who knew his job was to lead, empower, and minister to the new American people. He spoke to the common man. He spoke to high officials and wealthy citizens of the United States. He wrote letters to many royalty who lived in other nations and justified the uniqueness of this republic. He wrote compassionate letters of sympathy to others in times of grief (like the one above).

Logan Shannon is not George Washington (obviously). But can he have a profound effect at **this** point in **this** time and impact many people in entirely different ways? There's evidence of this by letters from just a few of many family members and friends. You can do the same thing!

But why a book about someone's letters? And why letters at all? Doesn't that take a lot of thought and time?

Letters are different than texting, instant messaging, facetime, or video conferencing. All these other forms of communication have their place, but nothing says more about a person's character or affection than when they take incredibly valuable time out of their schedule and hand craft a note or a long letter to someone telling them how much they care or apologizing when they are trying to make amends about a misunderstanding. It **means something** to the recipient of that letter! There was sacrifice. There was thought. There was an investment into that other person.

Does that mean every single document has emotions and mushy stuff slathered all over it? No. As we all know, collection agencies serve a purpose, but they don't write letters to people to start a loving or caring relationship. And then there are soldiers in the field who open a note with a familiar return address, and they expect support and hope from home. But open the letter, and you sadly find that a loved one has decided to end the relationship, striking into the heart at the toughest of all times.

My grandmother, Helen Kresser, wrote to my dad, Robert Kresser; during World War II; while he was fighting in the Pacific theater of war. My grandmother and grandfather probably averaged 12 letters per week! My father saved those letters and I have those letters to this day. Why did he save them? They were important to him! Why will I save them? They are important to me because they were about those that I knew! I have a record of what they were thinking as those brutal war-torn days went by.

Now here's a twist on the routine method of letter-writing:

This may sound funny, but what if **you could write *yourself* a letter,** what would you say? Many people write a journal or in a diary, and express the same things. So, how would you explain in writing why things in *your own life* have gone the way they have up to now? Could you encourage yourself to be a different and better person? Or would depression flood over you, thinking that nothing will ever come your way that would help your current situation? Would you plan to seek revenge because someone stabbed you in the back to get ahead? Or would you be so uncomfortable you'd just put the pen down or shut off the i-pad as the first thoughts came to you? For those who **_would_** write a letter to yourself, it would take some time; maybe a lot of time.

Many letters would have blurred ink from tears as different memories resurface. Many would have pauses due to taking time to laugh from a joke pulled long ago, and a prompt, quick, follow-up call to a long-time friend forgotten in the hurried flip of our calendar pages......

But our stories NEED to be told! Too many stories are buried under the personal piles of good intentions and misplaced

"Our stories NEED to be told. Too many stories are buried under the personal piles of good intentions and mis-placed priorities."

priorities. Someone has to step up and get it done. First, whose story do we tell? Secondly, "Who's going to make it happen?"

So it was with Logan Shannon and me. I was moved by his compassion, composure, and his spiritual comprehension. He is my friend, and I knew his story **needed** to be told. His story has been woven into the lives and onto the hearts of hundreds of people. But it hasn't been written down.... Until now. Logan has been written **about**. But now it's his turn.

So **how** will his story be told? How will we be able to tell what kind of difference Logan made so far in so many lives? We could ask his friends, right? Great idea! No GPS, microwaves, IM, or facetime. It takes TIME to create a well-thought-out letter with a message from one heart to another.

Many of Logan's friends stepped up, and invested that time to tell THEIR story of how Logan impacted their lives. We all know people in our circles of influence who fall into thinking that a disease, sickness, accidental injuries, or life-threatening situations is a dead-end road. Logan struggled a long time ago with the changes in his physical body due to his disease. It is a relenting condition caused by Duchenne Muscular Dystrophy. But he has accepted his condition as part of a greater plan, and Logan wants to share that with you.

So, in a series of interviews, Logan and I discussed how his life would touch the lives of hundreds, and maybe even thousands of people who are afflicted and those families who have a family member who is afflicted; and share a message of strength and hope that can change their way of thinking.

Logan has made a huge difference in this world, and those who know him know this. Because he made a difference in MY life, I wanted to help him get his message out to a world that's starving for authenticity and meaning. It is my privilege to work with Logan on this book, and to reveal the many letters both **to** Logan and **from** Logan in an inspirational collection that will touch your heart.

We want to invite you in to read our personal mail. We want you to peel back the curtains on some of his life and feel what we feel. Both Logan and I join our hearts together and extend ourselves to you. Ready to walk along this road with us for a while? Ready to laugh? Or cry? I thought so...

Lee Hamilton Kresser

Chapter 2

Logan's First Thoughts

You want to meet Logan? What's he like? Maybe one day, you *will* meet him. But in the meantime, how would you? Well, I sat down with Logan and found out a little on what he's like at this point in his life, and how he feels about meeting people.......

Lee: Logan, if you want to start a conversation with somebody, how do you do that?

Logan: Sometimes it's hard because of my elevation (seated in wheelchair and not standing) and because my voice isn't as strong as theirs. And it's obvious I can't shake hands because of my condition.

Lee: As you know, I like to shake hands. I do it as a sign of bonding, and I teach young people the importance of hand shaking the right way. But you don't seem to be hesitant to meet strangers, do you? You're not afraid to engage people in conversations, are you?

Logan: No. On occasion, I dealt with a lot of anxiety. I was kind of afraid earlier in life about speaking out and different things. But that's changed over time. I'm better now.

"Achieving goals has more to do with hard work than with intelligence. I didn't let my condition limit me, because it was one way to show that I was like everybody else!"

Lee: What about your high school achievement as a valedictorian? That required that you speak to a LOT of people.

Logan: The only thing I have to say about that is the achievement wasn't as spectacular to me as it was to others. Because in my eyes, more people are able to achieve that level than they realize. Achieving goals has more to do with hard work than with intelligence. I didn't let my condition limit me, because it was one way to show that I was like everyone else!

Lee: And with two brothers, you know guys sometimes like to roughhouse a lot, and you can't participate like they do. The physical part has constraints. But I'm sure there are ways that other guys can show their friendship like gently smacking you on the back saying, "Hey Logan, what's up?" Or if you're in lunch line or at a big game and your school wins, they'll maybe make like they want a high five. Tell me some other ways you can mess with your friends.

Logan: I can joke around with them like anyone else does. I don't see anything that I do as special. But I actually *use* my condition to mess with my friends or those around me.

- When someone in a crowd says, "OK everyone stand." I say, "Hey, that's prejudiced!"
- If someone says, "OK, everyone sit down." I say, "I beat them all to it!"

Lee: But some things might actually be special, even though it might not seem so to others. Like going from class to class in the crowded hallways. Some get bumped and shoved in friendship. Fellow students back in high school didn't form this wide clearing did they? Like a kind of "express lane".....

Logan: (Jokingly) Sometimes they mess with me by yelling, "Everybody, look out!" They'll turn around and see me. They'll realize it's just my friends trying to annoy me. They know I get a little irritated when I'm trying to get to class like everyone else, and they know I just want to get there without any special privileges. It doesn't happen very often, though.

Lee: Let's talk a little about school and the friends you had. OK? Let's go back several years when you were in elementary school. The funny thing about education in school, in particular we're talking about the combination of physical condition, home life, perception and belief systems.

And we get all these education experiences from school, home, church, and personal interactions. But if we talk primarily about school and we go back to possibly pre-school, kindergarten and elementary school like Clough Pike Elementary; can you explain what it was like as the disease began to take its toll?

Logan: I didn't really have the issues with fellow students as I did with other people. Most of the fellow students already knew how I started off and how it progressed. They remember me not being in a wheelchair and then having to be in one, so they were okay with it. They didn't treat me any differently than anyone else. So they see me for who I am. They remember me without a wheelchair so when I got a wheelchair, they didn't see any difference because they knew who I was before.

"They remember me not being in a wheelchair and then having to be in one, so they were okay with it. They didn't treat me any differently than anyone else. So they see me for who I am."

Lee: My granddaughter is close to the same grade as your younger brother Corey. Many times while I was at Clough Pike Elementary School to see my granddaughter, I would see the interaction with you and your family. It was special to see you supporting your brother. Have you ever been back to Clough Pike Elementary School since you have gone on to high school?

Logan: I haven't for a while. Probably the last time I went back to Clough Pike Elementary was when I was in seventh grade.

Mr. Brokamp was principal when I was there. He was one of my neighbors. It was a pretty big deal having our principal being our neighbor. It was really good to have the principal of my school completely understand the seriousness of my developing circumstances. It helped a lot. It's something to keep in mind how a principal needs to look at his students as important lives, every one.

Lee: Who was your favorite teacher at Clough?

Logan: Oh man! I can't really remember. They were all very nice people. They were really good. Clough Pike Elementary School was a very good school. Now that I think about it for a moment, it wouldn't be possible to pick a favorite teacher because they were all so good. Even the teachers that you didn't really like were still very good teachers. That's the kind of school Clough was.

Lee: You say you used to have a Bible study with fellow students who also went to Clough Pike Elementary School. Did you still have Bible studies with those fellow students even as you all went through high school?

Logan: Yes. I have maintained contact with many of my friends from Clough Pike Elementary. Joey Spiegel is one of my best friends still. Jessica Brenes is also one I have kept in close contact with. Carly Chafin is also one good friend that I have maintained from Clough Pike Elementary.

Lee: How was the administration at Clough Pike Elementary? Did they make you feel welcome as your condition progressed? Were they friendly and understanding?

Logan: We always got picked up and dropped off by our mom while we attended Clough Pike Elementary. Clough Pike teachers and administrators were always protective of children's innocence and did not tolerate profanity from any students while on property. One of the office administrators, Mrs. Little, even gave my sister Sydney her car when she sold it. So I can say the administration was very supportive on all fronts.

This first interview is done. Logan worked through the early stages of the disease with kids he knew. Everyone at Clough Pike Elementary School knew Logan when he ***could*** walk. Are you wondering how kids from other elementary schools reacted who didn't know Logan when the local elementary schools merged into the middle school? Well, they ***never*** saw him when he could walk. They were strangers to his situation.

These kids and teachers would be like you and me not knowing details about a person in a wheelchair and making assumptions before we get to know them. We eventually realize that any person is really WHO the person is, and not the body he or she is living in.

Logan was diagnosed with a disease that many of his class-mates weren't able to even pronounce. But they saw their friend, their classmate, their buddy slowly having more and more trouble with walking. So what was this disease? As you turn the pages, you'll learn more about Duchenne Muscular Dystrophy. Some of you may not have it, but may be struggling with something else. But for those who may not be familiar with it, you might like to find out more about that disease that those kids couldn't pronounce.

Chapter 3

Three Friends Speak Out About Logan

What are *your* friends like? Could they tell me something special about you that would fascinate me? Logan has many friends, and three of them want to tell you about him. These are friends that Logan has had over several years, and they have brought out some special reflections of how Logan Shannon has impacted their lives.

So many of us text now, right? But a thoughtful *personal* letter is really an art form. Some letters can be a single paragraph, some can be several pages. Have you ever received a 'piece of a person's heart' in the form of a letter that truly moved you?

Logan's life has changed dramatically since his diagnosis of Duchenne Muscular Dystrophy (DMD), a disease that slowly affects bodily muscles from functioning. Eventually, a person with this becomes totally dependent on others for even the most basic needs. They require mobility assistance like a wheelchair. But people around Logan act differently. Why? Because he is so positive!

Logan has many friends because he *is* a friend! These first three friends knew him when he was young and could still make it on his own. Then the ravages began to take their toll. But Logan didn't allow the disease to affect his friends or his outlook. It was that contagious outlook that brought people **to** him! Read how Logan's friends feel about him:

Macon Overcast has known Logan a long time, and wanted to share what he thought when he first saw Logan at a roller skating rink, gazing with curiosity as Logan would whiz around the rink in his wheelchair at about 8 miles per hour having as much fun as anyone there. He also talks about some interesting topics he and Logan covered during those years.

Jessie Brenes has known Logan since kindergarten, and wanted to express her feelings and memories. She knew Logan before he needed any walking assistance or crutches, and tells of how she would get real bossy about which of her fellow class-mates would have the opportunity to push Logan around in his un-motorized push chair. Jess also describes how she felt when she began to see the effects of Duchenne Muscular Dystrophy taking its toll.

Sam Becker has been friends with Logan since second grade, and has grown closer and closer to him as the years go by. He experiences Cerebral Palsy, and so his story parallels Logan's in many ways. Through their times as friends, they have leaned on each other as they cope with similar infirmities.

There will be more letters to Logan throughout this book, and all felt honored to write theirs. Logan knows the investment it took for each of his friends to do this for him and the readers.

First, from Macon Overcast:

Logan,

It has been eight years since we met at the Beechmont Roller Rink (near Eastgate area of Cincinnati, OH), and since then, I could not have asked for a more reliable and constant friend as you. I remember seeing you rolling around the skating rink **in your wheel chair**, going at a threshold speed of 8.5 mph, and feeling something subtly curious about you. I guess I enjoyed roller skating so much that I wondered how someone without skates would enjoy a roller skating party. I didn't contemplate you much, I just wondered. So, then I met you. It just kinda happened. I can distinctly remember two instances of you at that roller rink, but I'm not sure at which spot I first met you: I sat down next to you and Joey (a letter from him later in the book) on one of those round benches topped with purple carpet; or I hitched a ride on the back of your chair in the rink. After that, our friendship just grew. I struggle to remember any profound moments between us, but, when I think about it, that's why I love our relationship. We can just **be** around each other. We spent a lot of time chatting about dumb stuff and seriously discussing our hearts—some people have good friends because they do a ton of crazy stuff together, but us, we are just glad to have each other, and I know that when we either get down to talking about something serious or just goof with each other, a moment is hardly ever wasted.

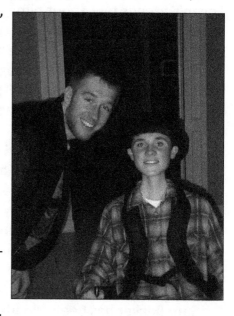

I know that you know, and you know that I know that you know me, and you know that I am curious about things that might not seem important to most people. But, I think you know that I am serious about wanting to understand things around me because you, too, understand that God values a person's experience. I know you are *sincere* in your pursuit of knowledge, and that's why your pursuit of God has given me an example that I can trust. I see the way you value your relationship with God, and through that, I can see the way you value your relationship with me. We are not so different from each other; maybe that's why I found you so curious that night at the skating party. I think our earnestness of thought separated us from a lot of other kids in high school because, while many kids search for answers, we held each other accountable in our earnestness before God. Like I said, not many people really appreciated our earnestness and looking back, you were one of the very few people that constantly valued me and my opinions. We could be transparent with each other, and that helped me develop a transparent relationship with God.

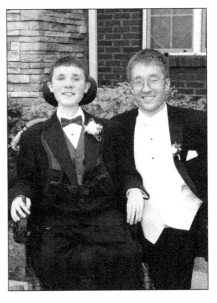

Among other things we were earnest about—girls. Goodness, it's like you were the fuse and I was the match. Combine us and we would explode into a forty-minute conversation about you and your latest love interest or me and my weird Facebook creepings. I think I told you at one point that I didn't ever want to get married. Don't worry about that now, friend, because I'm pretty sure it's going to happen. We may not be the "studliest" lady-killers around, but hey, at least we're honest with each other. Except with scary movies. We weren't honest with each other AT ALL about scary movies. I don't think any girl would have

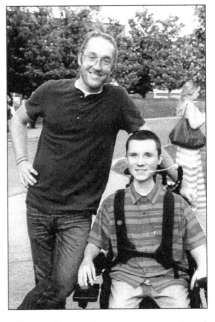

wanted to be seen within a mile radius of us when we watched our first four horror flicks. We were such cowards—I DON'T CARE

IF YOU SAY YOU WEREN'T SCARED WHEN WE WATCHED *LEGION*, WE WERE COWARDS! BE HONEST WITH ME HERE! After watching *Woman In Black,* I literally was scared of rocking chairs for the next month, and you even had a dream that your wheelchair did that same creepy rocking thing next to your bed! Girls don't want guys who are scared of horror movies. I think... I wouldn't know, though, so you might have to back me up.

Man, it was all about the time we got to spend with each other—all about the fun, relaxed, open, and honest time we spent together. It doesn't matter to me how we spent that time, whether in discussion, watching movies, or roller skating. I'm just glad we got to spend that time knowing each other.

In conclusion, we need to watch a scary movie soon.

Love you Logs,
Macon Overcast

From Jessie Brenes:

Dear Logan,

I was not a chicken! But there were advantages to having you as a friend who let me hide behind you and your wheelchair during dodge ball games at your church. In fact, there were many other times that you were in a protective mode for me.

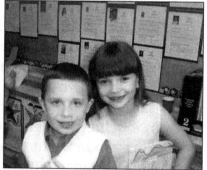

And it seemed as we went through our young lives that I grew into a protective mode for you over the years. Why was that? How did that happen like that?

I don't know if you do, but I still remember our 3rd grade class with Mrs. Ladenburger, and "Amber" and I would always argue over who got to push you in your unpowered wheelchair on any given day. We were both in competition for you, and you knew that, right? Although neither of us got to "officially" win you over, the good thing was that you and I later became BEST friends. In fact, the competition back in that 3rd grade class got to the point where the teacher had to make a chart for "turns" as to who got to push you in your wheelchair!

It's hard to explain why we could have so much fun and then wonder at the same time why you had to be the one to contract Duchenne Muscular Dystrophy. Why do some get sick and others don't? Or why do some students have such different attitudes when they get different diseases or injuries? It is always fun to laugh about those old times now when we look back at our elementary school days! You were different. As the years went on and physically your body was changing, you **_never_** changed. From the first day of kindergarten to today, you're still the exact same Logan that I've always known. And then when I think about it, knowing you and knowing your situation; and being your friend throughout all the years, you have changed *me*. Being that young and having a very close friend with Duchenne Muscular Dystrophy was hard to understand at the time, but I never seemed to look at you differently. To me you have just always been one of my closest friends that I know I can trust with anything and everything. Why would it matter if you were in a wheelchair? Why SHOULD it?

Our friendship sort of started the first day of kindergarten. The beginning of such a special friendship that will ALWAYS be cherished because not everyone is lucky enough to say that they've been friends after 15 years throughout elementary, middle, and high school.

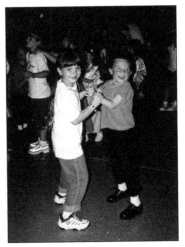

You were the very first boy that I thought was cute and had my first crush on. LOL. Not only did *you* know that but **EVERYONE** knew that. Why?

Because I wrote it all over my folders and papers at school, that's why!

I still have the notebooks full of notes with your name in the middle with scribbles all over it with words describing you and hearts drawn all over. And I felt so special in our middle school years when sometimes you'd allow me to ride ON your wheelchair. We were really close, and I remember us texting each other about our crushes! LOL. I remember when you invited me to go to AWANA at your church and we had a lot of fun! I also loved when you used to give me rides on the back of your wheelchair because you wouldn't let everyone do it. But you always let me... True friendship right there, right?

Looking back on our high school years, I think that's when I started really 100% understanding exactly what Duchenne Muscular Dystrophy was and how it affected you. And even when you were losing more and more muscle 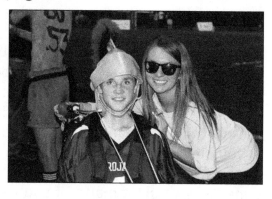 control, you kept on being the Logan we all knew and loved. You really were an inspiration to everyone around you. We had lunch together many times in high school and I always loved sitting by you so that I could help you and so we could laugh and joke the entire time! Why would we laugh and joke? Because you're hilarious and always making everyone laugh! You don't let DMD get in your way of living your life and it makes me so happy *seeing you happy*. Some people in your situation would give up and let life pass them by while sitting in guilt or sadness, but you are one happy guy. Maybe some of those people are afraid of what's happening. Maybe they don't have friends... But I think their feelings might change if they could have what you have. You have so many people that care about you and for you, friends and family that will always be here for you no matter what. And you know that God is real and will not bring anything your way that you can't handle!

You also inspire me to have a closer relationship to God because you are so devoted to Him and you just want everyone to follow! I'm sure I'm not the only one that you inspire, but throughout all the years I've known you, each year you teach me new things and every time I see you I can't help but smile because you're the strongest person I know. I am beyond blessed to be able to say that you are and will always be one of my best friends. We have so many memories and we could go on and on about them! Logan, thank you for being my friend for the past 15 years. You're the best! Love you Log!

Love,
Jessie Brenes

Letter from Sam Becker:

Dear Logan,
Wow, how do I, a person with Cerebral Palsy, begin writing a special letter to a special friend? The stories that surround both of us have to include wheelchairs, leg braces, air hockey, and that special embrace after **my first and only** varsity basketball game!

I know part of our story has to include that fact that we supported each other through our physical hardships; you had Duchenne Muscular Dystrophy and I had Cerebral Palsy. But our relationship didn't focus so much on leg braces and wheelchairs, it focused on being true

"I know part of our story has to include that fact that we supported each other through our physical hardships; you had Duchenne Muscular Dystrophy and I had Cerebral Palsy."

friends. Yes, we were both shy going into second grade, but that first air hockey game was the ice breaker to launch our friendship. At that point, I had very little knowledge of the effects of my Cerebral Palsy and I'm sure it was similar with you and your knowledge of Duchenne Muscular Dystrophy. In that, I think lies one of the beauties of our bond, we both see ourselves as if nothing is disabled **with either of us**. Because in truth, nothing is.

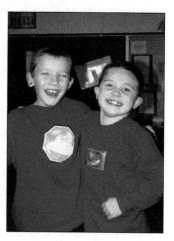

And who ever heard of TWO people playing first base at the same time for the same recess kickball team? I think the cool fact about that wasn't that we teamed up because we had disabilities, but just because we both liked playing the position and found it more fun if we worked together. For 25 minutes each day at school we were able to make our struggles disappear.

Remember when we were BOTH in wheelchairs for a while at Clough Pike Elementary School? Even though we were considered two of the more well-liked kids in our grade, I never really felt comfortable with my Cerebral Palsy when we were little. I was always embarrassed when I had those leg braces on, or would fall occasionally in the hall or out on the playground. I didn't like people asking me what was wrong, because I never really thought anything was. With the

"I was always embarrassed when I had those leg braces on or would fall occasionally in the hall or out on the playground.... With the exception of Trevor Jones, you were the only other person with whom I felt like I could be myself and not have to worry about my Cerebral Palsy."

exception of Trevor Jones, you were the only other person with whom I felt like I could be myself and not have to worry about my Cerebral Palsy. When I was with you guys, I never felt the awkward stares or that I was made fun of when I limped. After my surgery in 3rd grade my legs were so weak I couldn't even use crutches. So when I wasn't riding around in that wheelchair with you, I was using a walker.

I want to share this emotional fact: At no other time do I ever remember being made fun of so much as those days during elementary grade school. It was awful. People laughed at me and made jokes about my use of the walker and how funny I walked with it. Even worse; everyone but you, Trevor, and my older brother Max, kept feeling sorry for me. It got to the point where I didn't want to go back to school until I got my cast off and learned to walk again.

But things started getting better when I decided to be pushed in a wheelchair for the majority of the school day. Which means; I got to be **pushed alongside you** and **be next to you** during assemblies and other school events. Hanging out with you in our wheelchairs allowed me to get myself back in the flow of the real world and feel normal again. You helped give me something positive to take from a pretty negative time in my life.

"Hanging out with you in our wheelchairs allowed me to get myself back in the flow of the real world and feel normal again. You helped give me something positive to take from a pretty negative time in my life."

Going back a little bit, I'll never forget the first time we hung out going into second grade. I was really nervous because our moms just casually set up a play date for us and I didn't really know you at all at that point. I remember us both being really shy and exchanging little conversation (even though we both

love to talk). And during that first air hockey game in my base-
ment, after about a half an hour of playing, you hit this shot that
seemed to make the puck disappear in thin air. We looked at each other won-dering what happened to it. Neither of us saw where it went until I checked the goal and saw that the puck somehow went in. We both cracked up. Instantly, we both said it reminded us of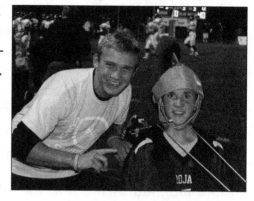
the final shot in the Mighty Ducks 2, which just so happened to be a mutual favorite movie of ours. And so the conversa-tions began!!

Immediately after we started chatting, I knew at that instant that you would become one of my best friends. It's funny how deep our friendship goes when it was started from such a childish moment. From that point on we seemed basically inseparable.

Some of my favorite memories were spent playing kickball with you and the guys at school recess. And it was so funny that we would always play first base ***together*** giving our team a little unfair advantage against the other. Nobody really complained about it either. It was the true beginning of our "tag-team" as we went further through life.

From the Mighty Ducks to kickball, our friendship has grown in so many ways. I have constantly tried to put into words the impact you have had on my life. Over the past few years, I have been asked to tell my life story to thousands of people. In each speech, article, or blog I have been asked to create, a section called the "Logan Shannon" section has been in it somewhere. That particular section has, and will always be, the hardest for me to write or speak about, but the most necessary.

At times, as I glance down at my notes during a speech and see your name, the tears begin to swell up in my eyes because I know I wouldn't be giving that speech if it wasn't for you. I have been called names like "Hero" and "Inspiration" so many times it makes me uncomfortable. So I apologize (but not really) when I say **you** are **my** Hero and my Inspiration. I know you are probably laughing right now because you always say I give you too much credit. Well I don't think so. I have never met a better person, a better friend, or a better follower of Christ than you. I guess that is why I have relied on you for the past 13 years.

God gave me Cerebral Palsy as my cross to carry, and He gave me you to help me carry it. You may or may not know, but I need to tell you this: each time I fell (physically or emotionally), you were there to pick me up and continue to help me push forward. Yes, I give God all the credit because He has worked through you to help make me who I am.

Throughout the next few years as our friendship grew stronger, unfortunately, your physical health declined, and mine has slowly improved. I can't really describe how difficult it was to see you confined to the wheelchair. I'd still do anything to trade places with you. To this day I wish I could have one granted wish from the "Fairly-Odd Parents", for you to be cured. At the same time, seeing you persevere and positively face your challenge head on was inspiring. From my perspective, the more you lost your physical abilities, the more you grew in your faith. And, as you and I both know, our life in faith and in God is much more important than our physical life.

Even when I had to switch schools around 6th grade, our bond remained as strong as it always has been. Sure, we didn't talk as much or hangout as much, but I knew you had a place in my heart, and I in yours.

Although you made an incredible impact on me during our grade school years, I believe it was our time at different schools that helped strengthen and solidify our friendship and helped me the most as an individual. My transition brought inevitable obstacles with me being away from my best friends.

Two of those major obstacles were 1) the heartbreak associated with my love for basketball, and 2) the embarrassment I felt when explaining my Cerebral Palsy to a whole group of people I didn't grow up with. When these challenges would crush my spirit, I could always look to you for strength and comfort whether you knew it or not. As the years went on, basketball (my favorite thing in the world), became harder on me. I was told multiple times that I would never play high school basketball and that I should try other sports like golf and swimming. Instead of quitting, I thought about you. Just as I would push you in your wheelchair you would push me through my workouts. People would marvel at my work ethic and determination on the court, knowing very well the physical struggles I endured. Quite frankly, my work ethic stemmed partially on how you thrived through Duchenne Muscular Dystrophy. No matter how hard it got for you, you always kept the faith in the Lord.

"I was told multiple times I would never play high school basketball and I should try other sports like golf or swimming. Instead of quitting, I thought about you."

That's something I wish I could say I did, but found I didn't. There were a few really tough times in my life where I questioned my faith. But you were the example to lead me out of the dark and point me back to the Light of Christ. You were, and always will be, my constant inspiration.

I want to let you know I wasn't going to step out onto that court on February 12, 2013 to play my first and only varsity basketball game without you in attendance. I thought about the game every day for four years. I visualized it before I went to bed at night and saw you there in the stands. I mean **you** were the one who pushed me through all my 5:00 AM summer workouts going into senior year. You carried me into the gym every morning without you even knowing, and every night to shoot thousands of shots, without you even knowing. Every rep in the gym that I struggled finishing, you helped me lift. Every step I ran each morning in the rain, sleet, or snow, you helped me make. I am not exaggerating anything or giving you too much credit, I'm just telling the truth.

The $3,247 I raised during the basketball game that night for the Cincinnati Children's Hospital Cerebral Palsy unit wouldn't have been collected without you. Why? Because the **Coach For Cure** event at Glen Este High School for Muscular Dystrophy inspired me to be part of the fundraiser at McNicholas High School's "McNick for CP". I wish I could've scored for you during my one-and-only varsity game, but I realize that the good Lord works in mysterious ways. I do not know why I didn't score despite my years of hard work, I do not know why I was given Cerebral Palsy, and I do not know why you have Muscular Dystrophy, but I do know it was for a greater purpose... **_For His plan_**.

*"I mean **you** were the one who pushed me through my 5:00 AM summer workouts going into my senior year. You carried me into the gym every morning without you even knowing and every night to shoot thousands of shots without you even knowing. Every rep in the gym that I struggled finishing, you helped me lift."*

As the final buzzer sounded in that game, everything was a blur. From the storming of the court, to being carried off by the McNicholas High School student body, and the swarm of hugs and tears that followed, all I could think about was finding you. As I finally found you through the crowd, my emotions took over and I physically almost collapsed. It hit me that it was just like when we were both in our wheelchairs in 3rd grade; nothing else mattered as long as I had you to help me and let me cry on your shoulder.

Thank you so much for supporting me and comforting me after the game. It was the only chapter of my athletic adventures, and I'm glad I had to carry my cross on the happiest, most emotional day of my life.

Thank you for always being there for me even now when I'm having a tough day or about to take an exam. Thank you for bringing me peace and faith in my abilities time and time again. Logan, I do not know what I would do without you and your Biblical perspective and encouragement. You are my biggest inspiration, my most trusted advisor, but most importantly my best friend. If I am blessed enough to keep on sharing my story and being an ambassador for perseverance, I will continue to speak of the invaluable impact you have had on me, and how your faith in Christ has helped me develop and grow as a man. Thank you for inspiring my family, and my friends, and people around the globe.

"Thank you for bringing me peace and faith in my abilities time and time again. Logan, I do not know what I would do without you and your Biblical perspective and encouragement."

As I try to be uncharacteristically brief in ending this letter, I just want to tell you I love you and I am so proud of you in all you have done with those around you and continue to do. Never have I met a more faith filled, selfless, loving person. I strive to be more like you every day. I hope I can make some small percentage of the impact on others that you have had on me. And in some way, I pray that I have helped you carry your cross, as well.

Love you, dear friend,
Sam Becker

So there are the first three. And there are more. But with these first three, you are almost in the presence of each person. We look into their eyes and we can see the reaction of what it's like to be around Logan. When we receive a letter from someone we know, we can actually hear their voice as we read it, can't we? Our relationship allows us to visualize their facial movements and actions. Letters from strangers are one thing. But from someone special, the hand-crafted creations are very personal.

Chapter 4

What is Duchenne Muscular Dystrophy?

Doctors have confirmed that Logan Shannon has a form of Muscular Dystrophy called Duchenne Muscular Dystrophy (DMD). You might have a different disease or condition that you are struggling with. It is tough. You might feel so down some days. And Logan can have those kinds of days too. You are not alone. Read on! So what is this DMD? How is it contracted? Who are the ones getting it?

Let's turn to the Muscular Dystrophy Association (www.mda.org) for its information:

Duchenne muscular dystrophy (DMD) is a genetic disorder characterized by progressive muscle degeneration and weakness. It is one of nine types of muscular dystrophy.

DMD is caused by an absence of dystrophin, a protein that helps keep muscle cells intact. Symptom onset is in early childhood, usually between ages 3 and 5. The disease primarily affects boys, but in rare cases it can affect girls.

What are the symptoms of DMD?

Muscle weakness can begin as early as age 3, first affecting the muscles of the hips, pelvic area, thighs and shoulders, and later the skeletal (voluntary) muscles in the arms, legs and trunk.

The calves often are enlarged. By the early teens, the heart and respiratory muscles also are affected.

What causes DMD?

Duchenne muscular dystrophy was first described by the French neurologist Guillaume Benjamin Amand Duchenne in the 1860s, but until the 1980s, little was known about the cause of any kind of muscular dystrophy. In 1986, MDA-supported researchers identified a particular gene on the X chromosome that, when flawed (mutated), leads to DMD. In 1987, the protein associated with this gene was identified and named dystrophin. Lack of the dystrophin protein in muscle cells causes them to be fragile and easily damaged.

*DMD has an X-linked recessive inheritance pattern and is passed on by the mother, who is referred to as a **carrier**.*

Diagnosis: *In diagnosing any form of muscular dystrophy, a doctor usually begins by taking a patient and family history, and performing a physical examination. Much can be learned from these, including the pattern of weakness. The history and physical go a long way toward making the diagnosis, even before any complicated diagnostic tests are done.*

CK level: *Early in the diagnostic process, doctors often order a blood test called a **CK level**. CK stands for **creatine kinase**, an enzyme that leaks out of damaged muscle. When elevated CK levels are found in a blood sample, it usually means muscle is being destroyed by some abnormal process, such as a muscular dystrophy or inflammation. A very high CK level suggests that the muscles themselves (and not the nerves that control them) are the likely cause of the weakness, although it doesn't tell exactly what the muscle disorder might be.*

WebMD (www.webmd.com) has some points to consider, as well. It discusses the different types of Muscular Dystrophy and we'll focus on Duchenne right now.

Muscular Dystrophy (MD) is a group of inherited diseases in which the muscles that control movement (called voluntary muscles) progressively weaken. Sometimes, the heart and other organs are also affected.

There are nine major forms of muscular dystrophy:

Myotonic, Duchenne, Distal, Limb-girdle, Emery-Dreifuss, Congenital, Facioscapulohumeral, Oculopharyngeal, and Becker.

Muscular dystrophy can appear in infancy up to middle age or later, and its form and severity are determined in part by the age at which it occurs. Some types of muscular dystrophy affect only males; some people with MD enjoy a normal life span with mild symptoms that progress very slowly; others experience swift and severe muscle weakness.

Duchenne Muscular Dystrophy (DMD) is the most common form of muscular dystrophy in children, DMD affects only males. It appears between the ages of 2 and 6. The muscles decrease in size and grow weaker over time yet may appear larger. Disease progression varies, but many people with Duchenne (1 in 3,500 boys) need a wheelchair by the age of 12. In most cases, the arms, legs, and spine become progressively deformed, and there may be some cognitive impairment. Severe breathing and heart problems mark the later stages of the disease. {End of WebMD information}.

So even with just reciting facts and strictly medical terminology per the above, Logan Shannon has bridged the wide gap in understanding *the condition of the body* and *who the person is* who has it. DMD affects the body mostly, not the mind.

Logan has shown that DMD is no match for the person. He has brought his brand of coping especially for YOU, the reader. We all know that the disease in the body will die when the body dies. But since the mind is a separate entity from the brain, the body will pass away, but who you ARE will not.

Through the years, Logan has brought healing to other people in ways that cannot be measured by blood tests, cat scans, or therapy. Even with physical restrictions that make things very difficult, he has been there for his friends; he has been there for his family, and he is now here for YOU.

The question is "WHY?" Because Logan cares. He knows in his heart that by reaching out and sharing his story, he will be extending his reach into the lives that need to hear a comforting word on those tough days. Let's keep reading to see what others say and let Logan speak to you again.

Chapter 5

Doctors and Medical Professionals

D o you trust your doctor? Of course, that's an easy question. Do you trust the nurses? Of course, they have extensive training, also an easy question. After some quick thoughts, Logan will speak about his feelings about his many medical issues.

Have you ever heard the expression 'The best patient is a well-informed patient'? When there is clear understanding, things go better. We trust our medical community because of their education, training and experience. When there is an honest and open discussion about our concerns, the best procedure going forward is determined. We actually feel good about that, even though it might not be exactly what we wanted.

So how do we feel about our medical experiences? Are we satisfied? In most cases, we know *any* procedure could have been worse. In this chapter, Logan brings his impressions together in a "letter" about the experience from his medical community. Also, two of Logan's physicians through the past years share their thoughts.

When we are not feeling well, or we begin to be suspicious about a soreness or lump developing in our bodies, we automatically turn to those who can offer answers and "make things feel better." During our early years, Mom or Dad would be there for us. In other cases, it could be an aunt, uncle or guardian. As we get older, we naturally turn directly to those in the medical field.

Have you ever written to your doctor and told him or her how much you appreciated an accurate diagnosis and recommended treatment and medicine? Normally we don't because we tend to be in a condition that doesn't lend itself to that. And when we get better, we forget until the next bout of sickness.

Ask anyone if they can remember when their doctor revealed a cancer diagnosis. I remember when my doctor told me that I had colon cancer. How many of us can recall when one of our loved ones had a serious accident and was in the hospital? Our emotions run high when we can't get any information. Have any of us felt that some in the medical field have more concern about the flesh of the body than the person themself? On the other hand, how many doctors and nurses truly reach out to their patients with care and understanding that makes us *feel* better?

Logan has been no stranger to hospitals, doctors, and clinical facilities. He wanted to collect some thoughts together in one letter about all of them. He has a simple and direct way of putting it in his own words. Even if you choose to pattern after this "letter" and put something in your own words to your doctor or caregiver, Logan would be pleased that you encouraged those around you:

Dear medical doctors & health professionals,

There are plenty of wonderful things that people in your avenue of work are doing, and I am very thankful for that. So now there are plenty of opportunities to ease the struggles that I suffer from with Duchenne Muscular Dystrophy. The medical system offers an extensive number of treatments and research into a disease as rare as DMD. I am very appreciative of this fact because I live in an area of the world and a period of time where I am privileged to have access to such things.

When I was younger I kind of took for granted just how much attention muscular dystrophy receives and how much help medically is available to those who suffer from it. So I feel the need to thank all of those who work in the medical field in general. Without anyone being interested in and doing work in this area there wouldn't be much help for anyone ailing from anything. More specifically, I want to thank everyone who had some sort of hand in treating, researching, and aiding in the progress of easing and curing DMD. One day, by God's grace, I truly believe that an end to muscular dystrophy is somewhere not too far around the corner. I hope that many people begin recognizing this and hop on board with supporting the cause.

But I will say, I think there are some things that can improve in the medical field: Initially, the expenses involved in all things medical are to me, far too high. I feel like the emphasis should always be on improvement of the quality of life for patients rather than payment of those offering their services. There should be more of you willing to truly be servants and sacrifice for the good of people as a whole than there are those simply in it for the pay. That's probably a war that those on the outside can't really fight, but I hope that gives you some food for thought.

Beyond that I feel like there needs to be much more availability of payment being met from different sources for those who constantly face medical expenses. I also feel as though there are certainly some doctors who could use some improvement in understanding what their patient's situation is. I don't have profound answers to these problems, but it can't hurt to share the concerns of those who on a regular basis deal with the health industry.

I also want to challenge those of you who are not medically, or financially, etc., involved with Muscular Dystrophy to get involved. In my opinion, it is one of the most, if not the most, difficult situations to deal with because of the wide range of physical limitations it puts on a person. Basically, every single part of life is 10 times harder than it needs to be (is for everyone else) for the ones with Muscular Dystrophy. Thankfully, there is amazing research going on for the condition and great progress going on in regards to the disease. Sometimes the medical community seems to be caught up more in supporting the improvement of a small handful of diseases that are far from being solved, and I think that it's important that the health community begins supporting the lesser-known conditions that have a ton of potential to be greatly improved in a much heavier way.

I hope that these words, from someone in my circumstance, are both a challenge and an encouragement to go deeper in your area of service and to do so with greater excellence!

Sincerely,
Logan Shannon

Here is a letter from Dr. Brenda L. Wong MD MBBS–Cincinnati, Ohio, who has been caring for Logan for years at the Cincinnati Children's Hospital Medical Center:

Dear Logan,

I can't believe I have known you since you were 5 ½ years old! It seems like a long, almost 15 years that we have been acquainted through Cincinnati Children's Hospital Medical Center's Neuromuscular Clinic. However, I really must admit I did not know you well until the last 2 years. I had not really understood the reason for your decision to stop steroids for treatment of your Duchenne Muscular Dystrophy in August 2006 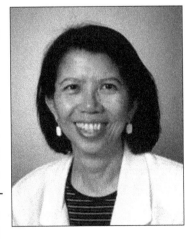 when you were 11 years old; and the firm decisions not to re-start steroids following your decline in your pulmonary function. It was not until I saw the video of your valedictorian speech and our encounter on that Christmas Eve a few years ago at my church that I started to wonder about your strong faith in a living God and focus on "things above and not of this world" that shaped your decisions regarding your care plans. If this physical life of ours is a pilgrimage and our destiny is for our eternal life, then our physical impairments and disabilities of our mortal beings are but temporal and should not be a big deal. You have encouraged my faith and I know you are a great inspiration to all who have met you. You have lived your life like salt and a light on this earth, touching many around you.

I want to say thank you for teaching *me* precious lessons of faith. Though your body is weak, your faith is so very strong and rises above life's challenges; so Logan, keep staying strong in your faith.

In His grace,
Dr. Brenda L. Wong MD MBBS
Director, Comprehensive Neuromuscular Center/MDA Clinic
Professor, UC Department of Pediatrics
UC Department of Neurology
Cincinnati, Ohio

Biography

Dr. Brenda Wong is a Professor of Pediatrics and Neurology at Cincinnati Children's Hospital Medical Center (CCHMC) and University of Cincinnati. Her specialty is in neuromuscular disorders with a focus on Duchenne Muscular Dystrophy.

Dr. Wong is also the director of the Comprehensive Neuromuscular Center and MDA clinic at CCHMC and leads an interdisciplinary team to provide integrated comprehensive care for patients with pediatric neuromuscular diseases and she is also active in clinical research and trials for patients with neuromuscular disorders.

Education and Training

MD: University of Singapore, 1980.

Residency: University Department of Pediatrics, Singapore, 1981, 1984-85; Royal Hospital for Sick Children, Edinburgh, 1985-88.

Fellowship: Child Neurology, Children's Hospital Medical Center, Cincinnati, OH, 1994-97; Neuromuscular Disorders, Hammersmith Hospital, London, 1997.

Certification: Child Neurology, 1998.

———

Logan also was under the care of Dr. Steven Agabegi for a time, and Dr. Agabegi is the surgeon who corrected scoliosis on Logan Shannon's spine by inserting two rods through his spinal column to straighten his posture. He wanted to share his thoughts on Logan in his letter:

Dear reader,

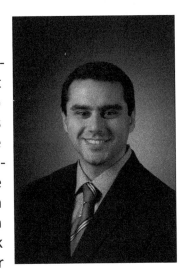

This is a short letter I prepared regarding Logan Shannon. I had the pleasure of treating Logan for his scoliosis several years ago. I did not want to make it too lengthy, and tried to keep it as succinct as possible. He has influenced many people, and I have learned a lot watching him, his valedictorian speech and the talk he gave on prayer that his father shared with me. He is an inspiring young man, I am so glad that you are putting this book together and I want to thank you for all your efforts.

I first met Logan when he came to see me for his spine deformity. Logan had been diagnosed with scoliosis several years prior, and when I saw him, his scoliosis had worsened considerably. My first impression was that of a very quiet young man, unusually mature for his age. I will never forget the smile on his face when I walked into the room, as he lifted his hand just enough to shake mine. As a teenager, receiving news that you need a major spine surgery can be difficult to take in. Logan listened intently to what I was telling him, he listened to the questions his parents asked and my responses to them, and that was it. I asked him if he had any questions and he said he did not. He was at peace with the news, with his condition, and himself. It wasn't a reaction you see in most 14 year olds. His surgery went well but he required bed rest for a week afterwards which can be very difficult after a major back fusion. Logan handled this better than anyone I have seen. Even my adult patients frequently have a hard time going through a period of bed rest after back surgery. Logan was not fazed by any of it. Over the last several years, I have had the pleasure of taking care of Logan and getting to know his family better. I have known Logan's father for many years. They are a wonderful family and have been blessed with this incredibly courageous young man. Witnessing how supportive his family is and how they rally around him in difficult circumstances is inspiring.

I realized later that Logan is a Christian. I watched his valedictorian speech at his graduation and it really did explain everything I had witnessed in my interactions with him. His quiet confidence and poise through impossibly difficult circumstances can only be explained by his faith. His speech was succinct and to the point: his faith in Jesus is what carries him. That's what it's all about for Logan.

Steven Agabegi

Biography:

Dr. Agabegi grew up in Philadelphia and graduated from Temple University. He then attended medical school at Temple

University School of Medicine in Philadelphia. He completed his surgical internship and residency in orthopedic surgery at the University of Cincinnati College of Medicine. He then completed a spine surgery fellowship at William Beaumont Hospital in Royal Oak, Michigan.

Dr. Agabegi treats all conditions of the spine, from the most straightforward problems to the most complex spinal deformities. He has special expertise in treating scoliosis and complex spinal deformities in adults and children. In addition to scoliosis, these conditions include kyphosis, flatback deformity and severe spondylolisthesis.

Dr. Agabegi is certified by the American Board of Orthopedic Surgery. His professional affiliations include the Scoliosis Research Society, American Academy of Orthopedic Surgeons and North American Spine Society.

Dr. Agabegi Education and Training

Pre-Medical Education (September 1993 – May 1997)
- Temple University, Philadelphia, PA
- Bachelor of Arts, Journalism

Medical School (September 1998 – May 2002)
Temple University School of Medicine, Philadelphia

Chapter 6

Mini-Letters From Logan's Peers

I asked several people who know Logan Shannon regarding how they felt about him. They responded very quickly with concise thoughts. These are their actual words, and I told them their comments could be anonymous, if they so chose. So some decided not to provide their names.

- "He is very passionate about what he believes in, and stands for. I admire him for that."
- "Logan is a light to our Singles Focus Church Group. He always smiles and keeps a great attitude on life. And he always wears hipster sweaters!" **Lauren Helton**
- "Logan is my favorite. And he is also my favorite 'beat boxer'. I love his sense of humor, and his comments are the highlight of my day!"
- "I appreciate Logan's outlook on life. He's one of the most real people I've ever met. He has always been super positive, and I've never seen him show anything but Jesus. And that's amazing!"
- "I think so highly of Logan because he is bold about his faith. I was inspired by his testimony when he gave it in church. Despite his circumstances in a wheelchair, he has

a positive attitude and his love for God is very evident. He is honestly a role model for me."

- "Logan Shannon is a spiritually mature Christian who has made a huge impact on me during my growth as a Christian. He has been one of those people for me."
- "Logan is the best ever!!!!!!!!!!!!!!! #Loganforpresident"
- "Logan is one of my close friends and an incredible role model. A lot of times, people are categorized by their physical abilities. People say: 'For someone who has gone through so much, he stayed focused on God and is such an inspiration.' But that's not right. Logan is an inspiration to me, and not because of what he's gone through. He's an inspiration because he's so much more focused on God's will than anyone else I've ever met. He is always someone I can look up to, and I know he's spiritually stronger than anyone I've ever met." **Greg Thompson** (love you, Logan)
- "I may not know you (Logan) really well. But I can tell you're really nice and always nice to everyone you meet. It's nice to know there are good people out there like you."
- "Logan's friendship with me reminds me of Jonathan's and David's friendship in the Bible. Logan encourages me, and is an inspiration to keep fighting the good fight." **Xavier Cortez**
- "Logan has had a very positive impact on my life. He is very happy to be serving the Lord, and you can see that happiness shine through everything he does. The last time I heard him speak publicly, I will never forget it. He spoke about God's grace, how God gives us His grace freely, and what that grace meant to him. I still do not fully understand God's grace. And honestly, it is not meant to be understood. To me, Logan is a living, breathing testimony of God's grace. I thank him for being the light as we Christians are called out to be."

Chapter 7

Adults Share How Logan Impacted Them

R andom comments about Logan Shannon by adults who know him:

- "I've only known Logan for a few years, but I'm very impressed by his attitude, his accomplishments and his love for the Lord. His positive outlook in spite of circumstances is a great challenge to me. I feel blessed to know him and I look forward to seeing what God will accomplish through his life and his testimony." **Andy Hendrigsman**
- "Logan is probably the most inspirational person I know. His faithfulness and love for the Lord has motivated him to use his talents for the Lord with extreme boldness. Serving with him has been a huge blessing." **Pastor James Neal** (Singles Pastor at Logan's church—www.fbcge. org)#loganforpresident
- "Logan is such a fun-loving, crazy man that I love to torment. And the spirit that Logan has exudes Christ as he shows general care for others. We all smile a little more being around Logan." Pastor James Neal's wife, **Kara Neal**
- "How can you not like Logan? He's smart, funny, and sarcastic in such a dry, funny way. He always seems to have a positive attitude. He is a reminder that we can always rise

above the trials that come our way." Church girls' youth leader, **Becky Bice.**

- "What can you say about a person who has suffered in pain most of their life and is confined to a wheelchair? You would think a word that would come to mind would be "sad". But it is my honor to just know Logan and see his always-positive attitude, love, and care for others with his wonderful spirit. I'm sure he has his low points, but he only presents his positive, loving side to those around him. What a wonderful person!" Church boys' youth leader, **Gary Bice**

- "I have had a lot of respect for Logan since the first time I met him. I didn't know him well, but I didn't have to in order to know he was a tough kid. He was always participating at school and in church activities. Once he came into our youth group, I became even more impressed with this young man as I learned his story. He has a heart for God and is always challenging others to grow stronger and have a bigger impact for God." **Joe Sherf**

Chapter 8

Intermission #1

Time to take a deep breath. Popcorn? Chips? Maybe you ***don't*** want to put this book down just yet. I can see why. Since everyone makes an impact in this world, **everyone**, read more:

Maybe you are really beginning to sense something about Logan. Time to get up for just a little bit to refill that cup of coffee, or get a warm cinnamon roll. The steam off the coffee and the contagious aroma drifting off that waiting pastry is simply preparing you for the anticipation of what the next "letters" may contain. Will these letters inspire me or not? Will

"Logan is also handing you a magnifying glass so you can peer deeper into some of his thoughts about what he's had to face."

these letters bring me hope looking at an uncertain future? Yet, you are realizing that there's really something here that will be of great value. If Logan could lift his arms, he'd reach out and place his hand on yours, and with a look of incredible compassion and understanding, would smile......

Look out the window. Do you see a busy street with the sounds of car horns barking for a position in traffic? Look around. Are you at the bedside of your child? Are you at the bedside of a parent? Do you hear the continuous beeps of hospital medical equipment launching audible notices to everyone in the room? Do you watch the drips of fluids into the arms of a loved one and wonder what's going to happen next?

Do you have visitors at the hospital or at your home to help share the emotional, financial, and physical burdens while caring for someone who isn't in condition to do it themselves? Do you feel like you're in an oasis where friends and family seldom drop by? With all that you're dealing with, go back to looking at Logan for a moment. How do others do it? How do parents of children, or children of parents, deal with the unexpected or continual burden of sacrificial caring? Is it love? Is it duty? Is it devotion? Is it just a routine? Is it because no one else will step up? Is it just a job? Is it something you choose to do to get by? There are so many situations that people just like you are in. Some days it may be love; the next day it could be routine.

At this point many of you have already been captured by Logan Shannon and are wondering how all these pieces are going to fit together. Hold on......... We're part of the way through now, and you've read letters from three friends close to Logan and some facts about the disease he copes with.

Logan is also handing you a magnifying glass so you can peer deeper into some of his thoughts about what he's had to face. When he started needing a manual wheelchair no one had an issue, as can be told by so many pictures. Why do these people feel this way? What is this that has created such a reaction from so many people? Who is this guy, really? Doesn't this make you want to know more about Logan? You may wonder how much more there is.

Do you wonder if he secretly harbors resentment about his situation and just wants to put on a front? Some may think so, and feel he has a hidden agenda to promote himself. On the other hand, some may see a person emerging from these pages that could inspire and encourage. Let's find out more about Logan to see if there is authenticity and sincerity in his character.

Going back to the letters from friends, many of us have friends to one degree or another; some close, some not so close. But could Logan maybe fall into the category of a great friend? Can a great friend just be a regular guy? It depends on what a regular guy actually is, doesn't it? But maybe he is so much **more** than a regular guy.

And Logan's in a wheelchair. Should that make a difference? Should seeing that mechanical mobility device make us feel differently? Does that make him NOT a regular guy? Could that be seen as a roadblock to a regular friendship or a relationship with a lady? So to clarify, Logan's **body** is in the wheelchair. His **mind** and his **heart** are not confined, but are alive and full of expectations, inspiration, and love!

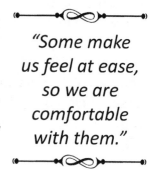

"Some make us feel at ease, so we are comfortable with them."

As we go about our daily routine, we associate with all kinds of people. Some make us feel at ease, and so we are comfortable with them.

These are the ones who will share lunch with you when you forgot yours. These are the ones who will bring a birthday gift when you didn't think they knew it was your birthday. These are the ones who volunteer to help on a last minute assignment that was dropped in your lap.

"Some people we know bring out disgust, envy, jealousy, and a whole host of other bad feelings."

Some people we know bring out disgust, envy, jealousy, and a whole host of other bad feelings. These people have burned us by spilling confidential beans to others and hurting our reputations and presence in our company, our school, or our church. They've lied about us so they can get ahead.

At work or at school, we know our bosses, our fellow employees, other students or teachers, friends or relatives that we naturally associate with, right? It's because we have things *in common* with them, right? Why? Because we *feel* relaxed and at ease with them. We all know the difference between spending time with those who lift us up and those who drown us in a swamp of drama all the time.

So what is it about Logan Shannon that affects people in such a positive way? Could it be that he *is* a great guy? Very possibly. Is he one of those guys who lifts us up when we're around him? Wait until you read some of the other letters......

If the only thing we could experience with another person was their voice, what do you think we could determine? Would we begin a conversation with them? Would we get disgusted right off the bat? Would we get a feeling of whether we'd like them or not? If you could hear Logan's voice, could you tell he was in a wheelchair? No.

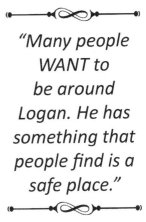

"Many people WANT to be around Logan. He has something that people find is a safe place."

After a great discussion, would you actually be surprised that he is in a wheelchair? Could it actually mean nothing that he's in a wheelchair?

Let's look at folks who are seemingly just like "us". Many disappoint us, and THEY are not even in a wheelchair. How many hearts have been broken and lives turned upside down because the person wasn't honest, wasn't sincere, or simply wasn't *there* for us when we were in trouble?

But here's the thing: Many people WANT to be around Logan. He has something that people find is a "safe place". Is Logan perfect? No. Even he will tell you that! As you read this book, carefully meditate on what is being said.

How about this: Dale Carnegie said, "You can make more friends in two months by becoming interested in other people than you can in two years by trying to get other people interested in you."

Logan IS interested in other people. He is that way. He has a heart for people. But is Logan interested in getting you to know him or like him just so he can feel good? No. I think that's the wrong question, from the wrong perspective. Logan is interested in showing you that despite really tough circumstances, there is something *more* to life than what circumstances show. I think the right question to ask is, "What does Logan have that people find so valuable, that they try to include him in their own lives?"

> *"What does Logan have that people find so valuable, that they try to include him in their own lives?"*

That would be a better perspective.......

So, if we looked in the rear view mirror of Logan's life, what would it look like? There would be pictures with family and friends playing or going to school. There would be vacations and road trips. There would be no hint of what was to come....

As the years ticked by, evidence mounted from Logan's walking and muscle control, a situation was developing. Pictures of manual wheelchairs were first, then motorized wheelchairs. But the friends stayed and circles grew. Logan's family grew as well.

The effects Duchenne Muscular Dystrophy would cause to the human body became clear. But Logan was not going to be held back by what he was riding in; he was going to live life!

Have a look at some pictures he selected to take you on a little journey through his life. On pages with the Wikitude app instruction, you can click on the page while holding your phone still over the page, and actually watch a slide show with many more pictures. Prepare to smile!

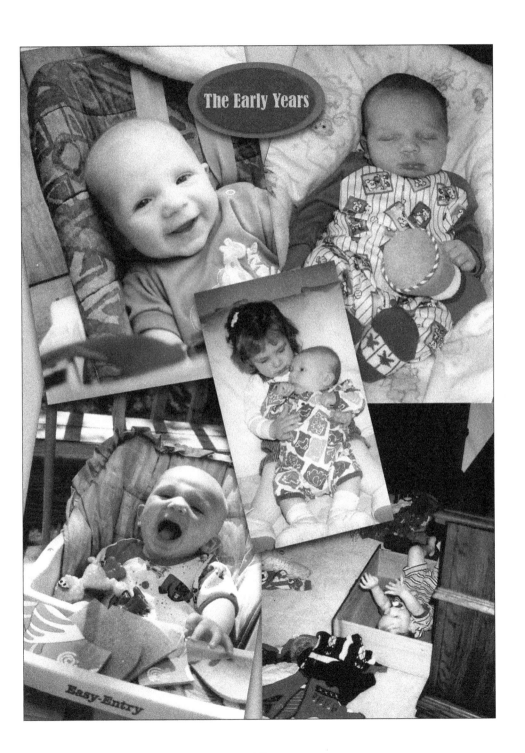

The Early Years

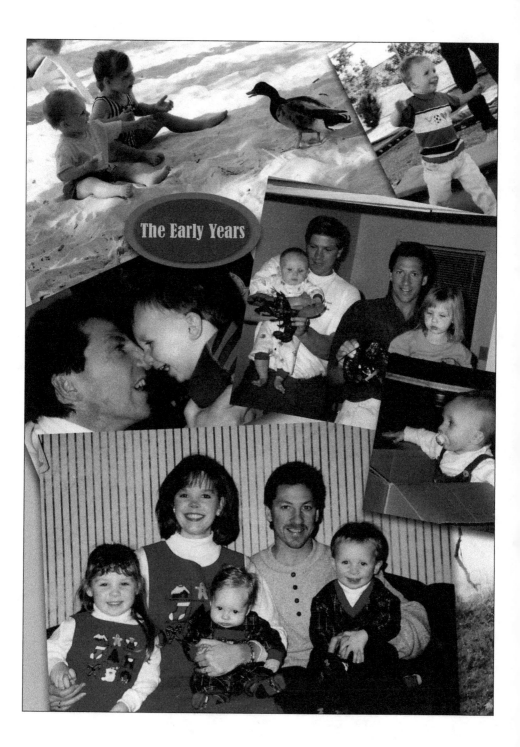

The Early Years

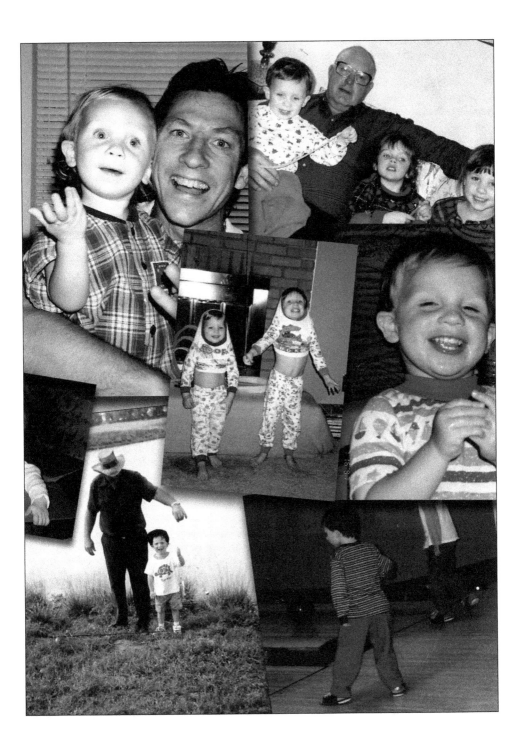

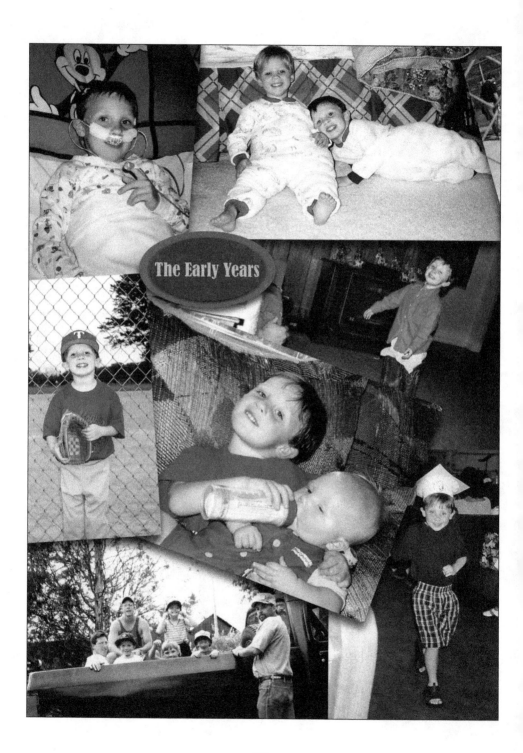

The Early Years

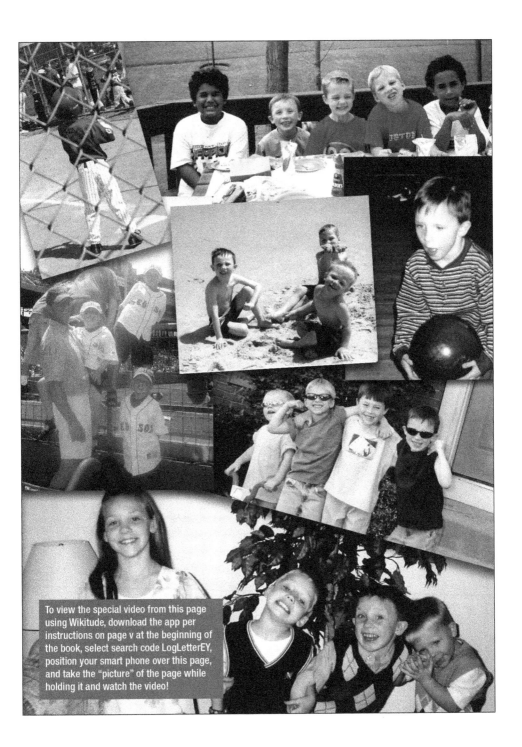

To view the special video from this page using Wikitude, download the app per instructions on page v at the beginning of the book, select search code LogLetterEY, position your smart phone over this page, and take the "picture" of the page while holding it and watch the video!

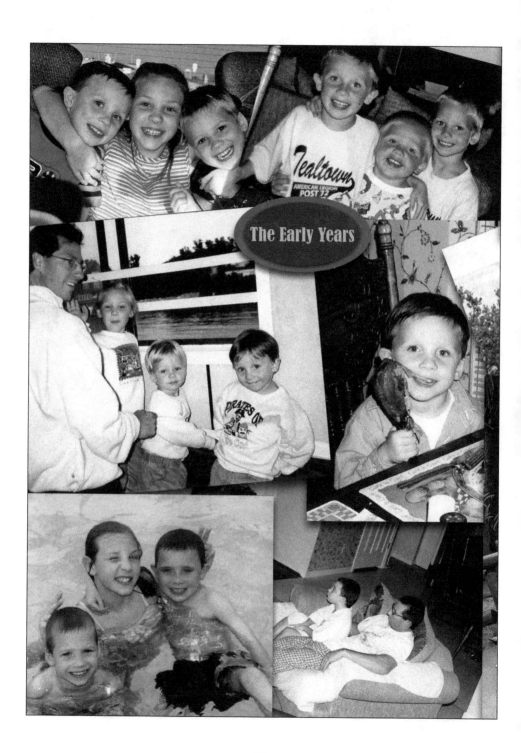

The Early Years

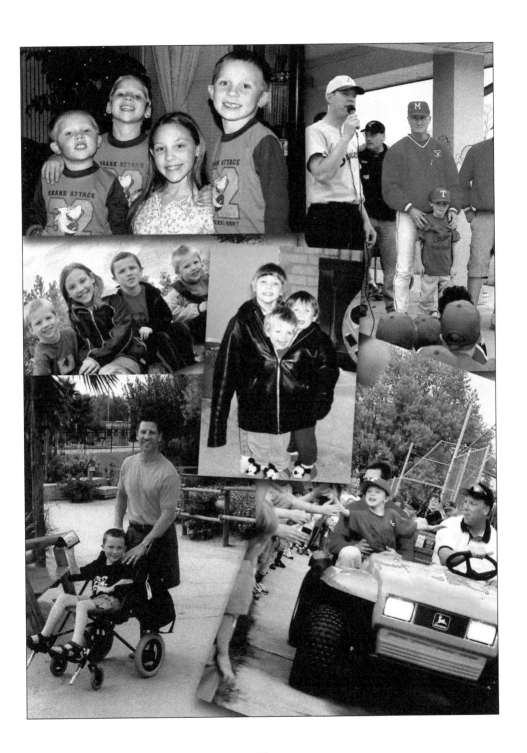

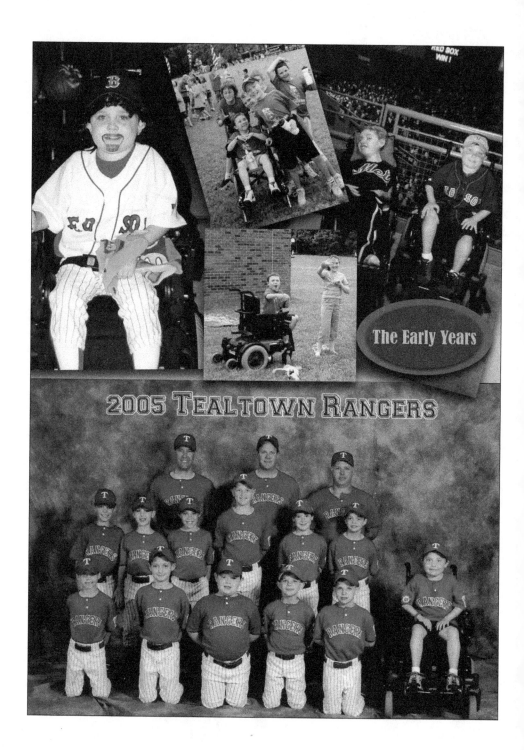

The Early Years

2005 TEALTOWN RANGERS

Chapter 9

I have Duchenne Muscular Dystrophy too!

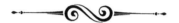

W e all know there are those who have dealt with serious ailments, diseases and conditions, don't we? We have experience in what that looks like. A soldier in the family who comes back with severe injuries, a dear friend who has cancer, or Parkinson's, or a close co-worker who had an accident on the highway.

Logan Shannon has Duchenne Muscular Dystrophy; there are many others who have it as well. Some are younger than Logan, some are Logan's age, and some are older than Logan. Both Tom

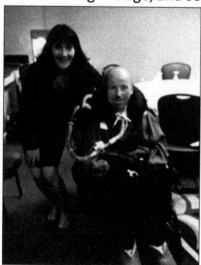

Sulfaro and Jonathan Fry have Duchenne Muscular Dystrophy.

Meet Tom Sulfaro. He lives in southern Michigan near Toledo, Ohio; and he wanted to offer his letter to Logan for this book. He is 43 years old, and his brother took Tom under his wing and has cared for him for years. Tom's brother also arranged medical assistance with a nurse who comes frequently to check on Tom. Here is Tom's letter:

Dear Logan,

My name is Tom Kevin Sulfaro and I also have Duchenne Muscular Dystrophy. All my life, doctors told me I would not live past 16. I know that without faith and hope in The Lord, I would not be here. I'm currently 43 years old! Lee Kresser has told me so much about you. He said you are 21 years old and confined to a wheelchair. He also said you have amazing friends and family supporting you. That says a lot! I wanted to write this letter to give you some insight into my life and how seemingly insurmountable tragedies can prepare a person for what will happen in the future.

First of all, "There's no such word as ***can't***." It might sound crazy. It might not be logical. But my Mom used to tell me that a long time ago. It was true then, and it's true now. And one key thing that stands out among many is:

I try to focus on all the things I <u>can</u> do.
"Don't wait to live!!"
So, where to start?
It's really easy to do: "God."

Let's do a little history first. When I was two years old, I was diagnosed with Duchenne Muscular Dystrophy (DMD). I was born the youngest of seven children and live in southern Michigan. Since I had an older brother with the same disease and five uncles on my mom's side, my mom knew what signs to look for. It seems like my mom was always taking care of someone else, and when she recognized the early signs, she

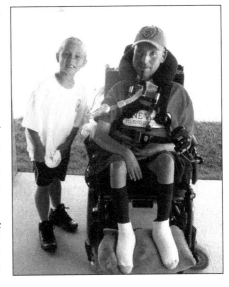

knew exactly what to do. Besides taking care of Frankie and me with DMD, plus five other children who did not have DMD, she also had to take care of my dad when his heart attack and strokes eventually left him incapacitated.

He was paralyzed on one side and practically catatonic until the doctors realized he was overmedicated. Her strength and perseverance were remarkable and I don't know how she did it. I recognize that there are so many people out there who are suffering from so many different diseases and chronic illnesses.

I sometimes think about these things, and KNOW that our heavenly Father knows each one of those families, and He is waiting for friends and family members to step up to encourage and minister to them, instead of dismissing them. Through ALL things, God makes good!

At the age of 16, my brother Frankie passed away from DMD. I was nine when he died, and my ability to walk ended shortly after his death. Because doctors told me I wouldn't make it past 16 and since my brother died at that age, I believed it. As my own 16th birthday approached, my fear of death became stronger and stronger. Even though she lost her son, it was my mom's unwavering faith and positive attitude that got me through it. God gave me one of the greatest gifts a person could get; a strong, faith-filled, selfless and loving mother.

However, three months before my 16th birthday, something horrific happened. My mom was tragically killed in a car accident. To say the least, my faith was severely tested. I was even mad at God. I thought, "How could He do this to me?" I also asked why God would take her because she was an amazing mother who took care of so many in the family. But eventually I realized that God has a plan for everyone and it's not for me to understand.

During this time, my siblings and I all pulled together to get through it and supported each other in a remarkable way. My faith grew stronger; enough even to forgive the man who caused the accident. This was not easy, but with God, all things are possible.

Immediately after the accident, my 21-year-old brother, Bob, took the lead as my primary caregiver since my dad was unable to. I'm so amazed at how selfless he was then, and still is. About four months after my mom's death, I ended up in the hospital with a double pneumonia. I almost died twice. During the second near-death experience, my mom appeared to me and she told me everything would be OK. Obviously, another gift from God to comfort me. The doctors gave up on me but my siblings begged someone to help. God heard their cries and a nurse stepped up and told them I could go on a ventilator to help me breathe. Looking back, God must have told her to speak up or maybe she was an angel. Either way, I lived past 16. I came home after a five-month battle in the hospital. I am so thankful that my brother, and best friend, Bob, continues to care for me. God has blessed me with the most amazing, loving and caring brother. We live together in a house and we have had a count-less number of excellent nurses over the years to help us out... another gift from God.

Logan, this may be hard to believe, and although DMD patients often get sick, I went twenty five years without being admitted to the hospital again. About four years ago, I found out that my heart was also greatly affected by my disease. However, with medication and God, my heart has dramatically improved. Although I'm in constant pain from my severe scoliosis and dete-riorating muscles, the Lord has shown me how to deal with it and has given me a high tolerance for pain. I try not to complain, however, this may unintentionally mislead others into thinking I don't have a terminal disease. In addition, I don't complain just to remind them of it, either. On some of those tough days, I wonder "why me?", but then I count my REAL blessings and say "why *not* me". I try not to feel sorry for myself. I have come to realize that my circumstances and struggles have shaped me into who I am today. I wake up every day thankful to be alive and I get out of bed regardless of how I feel.

I also told you before that one of my mom's favorite sayings was "there's no such word as can't." She made me believe that nothing is impossible. Since I try to focus on all the things I *can* do instead of what I ***can't***, I've men- tored patients and families, done some public speaking, and some fundraising for my disease. Who knew that over the years I'd be involved with all that?

I enjoy visiting with friends and family, playing cards, going to the movies, and out to eat. My brothers and I have a passion for cooking, and boy can we cook! Thank God I can still eat. I am on Facebook and have over 200 "friends" connected to Duchenne. I also started a social group in our home of DMD patients and their families in order to share our stories and struggles.

This continued until about 3 years ago when my good friend, Brian, who attended the group, passed away. Since his passing, I've had a hard time keeping it going. I hate it when someone dies from this disease.

Sometimes I don't always see it, but I know that God loves me and has a purpose and plan for my life. I have discovered that mine is to help others by giving them hope and encourage- ment to push through any obstacle, and to live life regardless of this or any dreadful disease, or whether or not there's a cure. Remember: ***Don't wait to live.***

I have found so much inspiration from Duchenne patients older than me on Facebook. I only hope that I can be an inspira- tion to you, Logan. Find your purpose. You can be an inspiration to someone else.

God bless you Logan,
Tom

Jonathan Fry is Logan's age and lives in west central Florida, and I had a chance to meet him while I was visiting his church there. This 23-year-old guy was sharp, had a great smile and personality, and even looked a little bit like Logan. Here is the letter he offered to write to Logan:

Dear Logan,

My name is Jonathan Fry and I have DMD like you. I was diagnosed when I was only 3 years old and cannot remember a time when I thought I would be the same as everyone else. I endured slowly losing my ability to walk until finally I was confined to a wheelchair at age 12. I've gone through spinal fusion surgery to correct scoliosis in my back and hospital stays as a result of heart and respiratory issues.

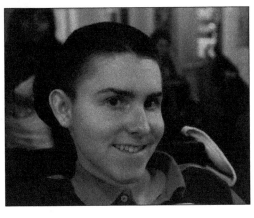

It would be un-surprising if I was bitter and depressed as a result of all these things. However, my faith in Jesus Christ as my Lord and Savior has filled me with what can only be described as a supernatural hope and peace that cannot be extinguished. The promises that are in God's Word are what keep me going. My favorite Bible verse will always be Philippians 4:13 – "I can do all things through Christ who gives me strength." (NIV)

Through all of life's hills and valleys, it is imperative to remind ourselves that Jesus will provide us the strength we need to get through the challenges that we face. The ups and downs of my life have taught me many lessons over the years. Growing up, I was involved in a program called AWANA which stands for Approved Workmen Are Not Ashamed. AWANA is a program in which pre-school through grade school children memorize Bible verses and recite them to adult leaders in pursuit of certain rewards. AWANA taught me the importance of knowing Scriptures that you can recall when dealing with temptation or physical limitations.

A secondary part of AWANA is "game time" when kids get to play group games to get out some of their abundant energy. It was there, when I was 12, that I had one of the wildest experiences of my life. I was in a manual wheelchair at that point and couldn't participate in a game which involved running from one end of the gymnasium to the other.

The father of one of my friends wanted to get me involved and told me to buckle my seat belt, which I did. He then proceeded to push me as fast as he could, keeping pace with the fastest kids. As we approached the padded wall, I began to yell at the top of my lungs in a crazy combination of fear and exhilaration. But he slowed down in enough time and the front of my chair softly touched the padded wall. After catching my breath, I realized how much fun that was and asked him to do it again. He did that plenty of times in the next few months, and we still joke about that to this day.

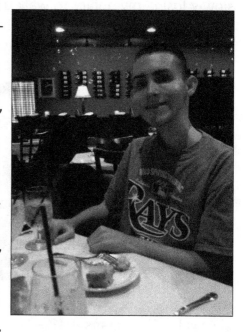

At the same time, my life has not been devoid of frustrations. As my muscles have gotten weaker, I've had to learn how to adapt to that. It's irritating to have to adjust the way I do things to compensate for my lessening abilities. On the other hand, my mother pointed out that it is an opportunity to learn something new. This process, although difficult, has taught me perseverance.

Additionally, my relationships with other people have been affected by DMD. There was a girl I met while attending college who was going through a tough breakup with her boyfriend. As

I listened to her problems and encouraged her over the next couple of weeks, we became friends. She was the first girl I was friends with in 4 years and after about six months of being friends I started entertaining thoughts of dating her. But I was far too nervous to ever say anything and she never considered me to be someone who she could date. We've since lost contact with each other after she stopped attending college.

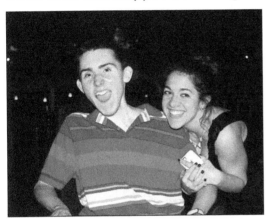

I am sometimes tempted to be bitter about this situation I am in, but I look to the Bible when that happens. Paul, in 1 Corinthians 7:26-27, says "I think that it is good for a man to remain as he is. Are you pledged to a woman? Do not seek to be released. Are you free from such a commitment? Do not look for a wife." (NIV) Although this verse is often hard for me to accept, I know that a relationship with the Lord will bring me far more pleasure than getting married will. Through the good and the bad, my faith in Jesus is the cornerstone of my life. 1 Timothy 1:19 tells us to "Cling to your faith in Christ." We must remind ourselves that He is always with us and will carry us through life, no matter how big the obstacles are. Stay firm in the faith.

Your brother in Christ,
Jonathan Fry

Chapter 10

"We have wheels too, and we kept going!"

We're in wheelchairs too and that doesn't stop us! What about Joni Eareckson Tada, who overcame so many obstacles as a Christian quadriplegic? What about Gerry Bertier (from a story and football-themed movie made about 15 to 20 years ago)? He was able to overcome his paralysis, as well.

We'll let Joni Eareckson Tada express her heart first. Then we'll read about Gerry Bertier and his successes after that terrible car crash that paralyzed him.

Joni was in a diving accident when she was a teenager, and has been in a wheelchair since 1967, she sent the following letter to Logan.

Dear Logan...

Recently I learned the details of your story and that you have been dealing with Duchenne Muscular Dystrophy for all your life – and it's why I had to put down everything and write you right away. Because of my own disability, I know how uplifting it is to receive words of encouragement; after all, the Bible

"Because of my own disability, I know how uplifting it is to receive words of encouragement..."

tells us to "encourage one another daily" (Hebrews 13:3). And often just a little encouragement from a fellow journeyer can go far...

Because, Logan, after 47 years of living as a quadriplegic in a wheelchair, there a*re st*ill mornings I wake up and th*ink, I can't go on; I don't have the strength.* It's the way the apostle Paul felt in II Corinthians 1:8-9, *"... We were under great pressure, far beyond our ability to endure, so that we despaired even of life..." (NIV)* (I'm **sure** you've felt like that). Yet the next verse provides such hope: *"But this happened that we might not rely on ourselves but on God."*

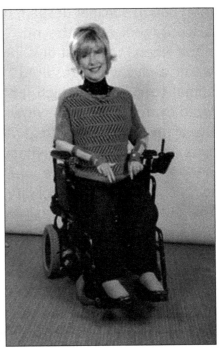

Logan, *that's* the secret to moving on with life. The weaker we are, the harder we must lean on Jesus; and the harder we lean on Him, the stronger we discover Him to be. So for all the struggles that DMD will throw at you in the weeks and months to come; for all the mornings you'll wake up and need courage, I'm praying Colossians 1:11 from *The Message: "We pray that you will have the strength to stick it out over the long haul–not the grim strength of gritting your teeth, but the glory-strength God gives. It is strength that endures the unendurable and spills over into joy, thanking the Father who makes us strong enough to take part in everything bright and beautiful that He has for us."* Yes, may God's courage be yours. And God bless you for the way you spread His courage to others through your upbeat, positive outlook on life – your joy is contagious and that makes you a wonderful ambassador for the Gospel, dear Logan. May you know the nearness of God today!

Yours in His care,
Joni Eareckson Tada (pronounced "Johnie")

An excerpt and partial bio from The Joni Eareckson Tada story, from her website **www.jonieareksontadastory.com** : As a teenager, I loved life. I enjoyed riding horses, loved to swim. It hardly seems 26 years ago, that I was lying on a hospital bed in suicidal despair, depressed, discouraged, after the hot July afternoon when I took that dive into shallow water, a dive which resulted in a severe spinal cord injury, which left me paralyzed from the shoulders down, without use of my hands and my legs. Before that time, I didn't even know what you called people like me. **Who are we?** The physically challenged, the mobility impaired, the differently-abled, handicapped. I knew we weren't crippled or invalid. But

"I could not face the prospect of sitting down the rest of my life without the use of my hands, without the use of my legs. All my hopes seemed dashed. My faith was shipwrecked."

I just didn't have any contact with people who were hurting or in pain. That seems to be a common topic these days and many of the disabled people that I know even in the nineties have a tough time finding life worth living. I sought to find a final escape, a final solution, through assisted suicide, begging my friends to slit my wrists, dump pills down my throat, anything to end my misery. The source of my depression is understandable. I could not face the prospect of sitting down for the rest of my life without use of my hands, without use of my legs. All my hopes seemed dashed. My faith was shipwrecked.

I was sick and tired of pious platitudes that well-meaning friends often gave me at my bedside. Patting me on the head, trivializing my plight, with the 16 good Biblical reasons as to why all this has happened. I was tired of advice and didn't want any more counsel.

"I was tired of advice and didn't want any more counsel. I was numb emotionally, desperately alone, and so very, very frightened."

I was numb emotionally, desperately alone, and so very, very frightened. Most of the questions I asked, in the early days of my paralysis, were questions voiced out of a clenched fist, an emotional release, an outburst of anger. I don't know how sincere my questions really were. I was just angry. But after many months, those clench-fisted questions became questions of a searching heart. I sincerely and honestly wanted to find answers.

Now I knew, in a vague sort of way, that answers for my questions about my paralysis were probably hidden some-where between the pages of the Bible, but I had no idea where. I needed a friend who would help me sort through my emotions, who would help bring me out of the social isolation, who would help me deal with the anger. A friend who would point me somewhere, anywhere, in God's Word to help me find answers. I found a friend, a young man named Steve, who knew absolutely nothing about emptying leg bags or pushing wheel chairs and he had no idea what to call people like me, whether we were physically challenged, differently-abled, mobility impaired. Don't you get tired of all those fancy, schmancy euphomisms?

I remember my friend Steve, just a young teenager, who had a caring, compassionate heart, a love for God, and a halfway decent working knowledge of

"I needed a friend who would help me sort through my emotions, who would help bring me out of social isolation, who would help me deal with the anger. A friend who would point me somewhere, anywhere, in God's Word to help me find answers."

the Bible. At my bedside, I cornered him one day, and I said to Steve, "I just don't get it! I trusted God before my accident. I wasn't a bad person. This couldn't possibly be a punishment for any sin that I've done. At least, I hope not. I don't get it, Steve? If God is supposed to be all loving and all powerful then how can what has happened to me, be a demonstration of His love and power?

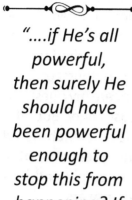

"....if He's all powerful, then surely He should have been powerful enough to stop this from happening? If He's all loving, then how in the world can permanent and lifelong paralysis be a part of His loving plan for my life? I just don't get it! Unless I find some answers....."

Because, Steve, if He's all powerful, then surely He should have been powerful enough to stop my accident from happening? If He's all-loving then how in the world can permanent and lifelong paralysis be a part of His loving plan for my life? I just don't get it! Unless I find some answers, I don't see how this all loving and all powerful God is worthy of my trust and confidence. Who is in control? Whose will is this anyway?" I said to him.

My friend Steve took a deep sigh and he was wise enough to discern that my question, again, was not voiced out of clench fist, but out of a searching heart. He knew I sincerely wanted to find an answer. And so he said, "Joni, those are tough questions, and theologians have been trying to answer them for hundreds of years. I can't pretend to sit at your bedside and know why and how.

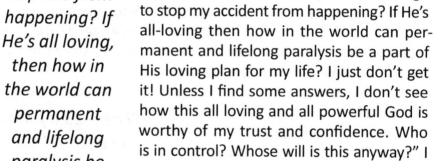

I can't pretend to explain the loving nature of God and how your accident is a demonstration of His power. But when it comes to the question about who is in control, and whose will is this anyway, I think I can show you some answers." Huh, well! I wanted to see this! So I waited to see what he would say. I thought he might quote to me the 16 good Biblical reasons as to why all this has happened.

Joni shares a lot more on her website:

www.joniearecksontadastory.com

But here are a few more comments from the whole text:

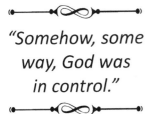

"Somehow, some way, God was in control."

Somehow, some way, God was in control. I am convinced that God's motive, God's purpose, His plan in the accident in which I became paralyzed, His purpose was to turn a head-strong, stubborn, rebellious kid into a young woman who would reflect something of patience, something of endurance, something of longsuffering.

Who would get her life values turned from wrong side down to right side up and would have a buoyant and lively optimistic hope of heavenly glories above.

I wouldn't dare list 16 good Biblical reasons as to why this accident happened to me. No I wouldn't dare do that because suffering is still a mystery. I can't explain it all and my friend Steve couldn't explain it all by my bedside either. It's a mystery, but not a mystery without direction. We know for one thing in this mystery, nobody is glorifying suffering. God does not think this, that a spinal cord injury is a great idea. There is no inherent goodness in cerebral palsy, muscular dystrophy, multiple sclerosis, cystic fibrosis,

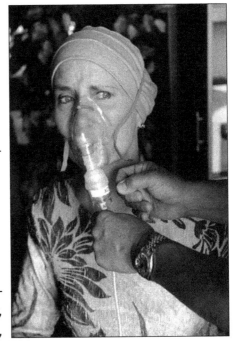

brain injury, stroke, heart disease, manic depression, No, No, No! There is no inherent goodness in disease or disability; but like I said, God can reach down to what would otherwise seem like a terrible difficulty and wrench out of it positive good for us and glory for Himself. There is no inherent goodness in disability, disease, or deformity but we are promised in the book of Romans the 8th chapter, the 28th verse that all things can fit together into a pattern, a plan for good, our good and His Glory.

"God used this injury to develop in me patience and endurance and tolerance and self-control and steadfastness and sensitivity and love and joy. Those things didn't matter much when I was on my feet but, boy, they began to matter after I began living life in a wheelchair."

I remember when my friend Steve shared that verse with me as well, and I challenged him saying, "That sounds to me that you're saying, there, that all things are good." He said, "No, Joni, that's not what the verse says. It doesn't say that all things are good. It just says that all things can fit together into a pattern for good, a plan for good."

God used this injury to develop in me patience and endurance and tolerance and self–control and steadfastness and sensitivity and love and joy. Those things didn't matter much when I was on my feet but, boy, they began to matter after I began living life in a wheelchair. For one thing, the Bible assures us that we're going to have new bodies. First Corinthians, chapter 15, read it sometime for some encouragement. We learn there that one day we will have new hands, new legs that will walk, new hearts, new minds.

I can't pretend to know all the answers, honestly. But I know what has worked for me from God's Word. I know that God's

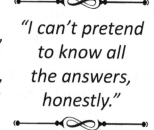

"I can't pretend to know all the answers, honestly."

Word can come alive and active in your life as well. You see, the choice is yours. That's what's given it new meaning, new hope, new victory. The same is true in your life as well. This wheelchair to me use to symbolize alienation and confinement, but God has exchanged its meaning because I trusted in Him. Now this wheelchair to me is a symbol of independence and freedom and mobility. It's a choice I made and it's a choice you can make too. You won't

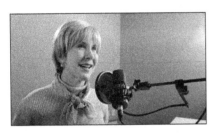

be able to make it overnight some of you. It will be a long hard haul for a few of you. There will be dark days when you will ask questions, not out of a searching heart but you'll voice them out of a clenched fist, but that's ok. God is big enough to handle our biggest doubts and He's not held hostage by our handicaps. Oh, no, He cares and He welcomes all the doubts, the fears, the questions, and the frustrations. The grace is His, the choice is yours. Would you let Him reach down into an otherwise, seems to be awful pain in your life and wrench out of it positive good for yourself and glory for Him.

"Father, thank you so much for the Lord Jesus Christ who died on the cross for me. I confess my rebellion, pride, stubbornness. I lay it all at the foot of the cross. Father, I thank you that Jesus has paid the penalty. You have no more anger left for me, only love and mercy. I receive that love and mercy now as I confess my sin. Thank you that Jesus is my Savior and I bless you for the difference He will make in my life. Help me to follow you in the power of His Spirit. In Jesus name, Amen."

I face a lot of limitations what with living in a wheelchair for over 26 years, but I have found limitless joy and peace in knowing the Lord Jesus. I want you to know I really care for you and your spiritual walk. God bless you on your spiritual journey.

———◆———

Remember Gerry Bertier, who wore #42, and whose character was shown in a movie made about 15 to 20 years ago?

You may or may not remember, but it was a cool football movie (no matter what liberties Hollywood took in making it). It is a real story of a high school football team that was born out of a consolidation of other schools and their respective programs. Gerry Bertier was cast as one of the actual football players by an actor in the movie. The movie portrayed Gerry Bertier being in a car accident, and that was true. Despite being in a wheelchair from those injuries, Gerry went on to be a very productive citizen and positive contribution in the lives of many. How many of us expect something different? Would we think that people in wheelchairs cease to become inspirational? Does this mean their passion disappears or their purpose in life disappears? Gerry lived his life until April 20, 1981, when a drunk driver crossed the median and hit Gerry's car head-on. This time, Gerry didn't make it.

A foundation has been set up for him where spinal research can continue. Please consider donating! **Gerry Bertier 42™** is a registered trademark. But here is more about Gerry from the website set up for him <u>www.gerrybertier.com</u> :

The Early Years

Gerry William Bertier was born August 20, 1953, and was raised in Alexandria, Virginia. Gerry was raised mostly by his mother, Jean. Mrs. Bertier watched her son grow up to be a happy and successful young man. During Gerry's childhood he had mentioned being in the Olympics. His long-term goal was to receive a gold medal. Gerry aged and entered into his high school years. He blossomed as an athlete and

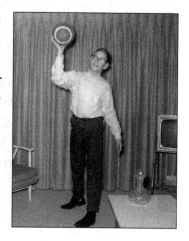

by his senior year, he starred in football, basketball and track, eventually ending up at T. C. Williams High School as part of the desegregation of three schools. Hammond High School was the school he previously attended. At T. C. Williams, he quickly became involved with the football team.

Things were quite rough in the beginning, but through the struggle and cooperation of his fellow teammates, the Titan team made it through a "perfect" no-loss season. The team set the school on fire, routing one opponent after another. T.C. Williams marched to the state title, and afterward, Gerry Bertier, the team's 6-foot-1, 200-pound roughneck linebacker, reaped the fruits of a remarkable season: He was named one of the top 100 high school football players in the nation and voted All-Everything from All-

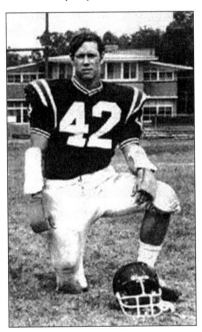

American on down, and he was offered many scholarships, including ones from Alabama and Notre Dame.

It was quoted in the Richmond News Leader, Dec 1971 issue that as a linebacker, "Gerry threw opposing backs for 432 yards in losses-52 yards more than were gained net against the state champions. Bertier was credited with 142 individual tackles, including dumping opposing quarterbacks 42 times." I doubt Gerry had any idea what great things he was about to enter into, nor do I believe he had any idea how his athletic participation would make such an impact in Alexandria, Virginia sports history. To clear up any misconceptions that the movie might have left in the viewer's mind, Gerry did not have his football success come to an end until after the state championship.

"Life Is Not Over"

The night of the football banquet dinner, December 11, amid warm, enthusiastic applause, Gerry was awarded the team's Most Valuable Player trophy. Gerry was on top of the world. Then tragedy struck. That fateful night after the banquet dinner, Gerry rounded a curve only two blocks from his Alexandria home, he and his mother's new Camaro ended up in a terrible accident which caused his paralysis. The cause of the accident was later deemed to be a mechanical failure in the motor mount of his engine.

Almost immediately, Gerry accepted his paralysis and vowed to live a productive life. Doctors figured he might remain in the hospital for almost two years. But a month and a half after the accident, he made a temporary exit. Driven by ambulance, rolled in on a stretcher

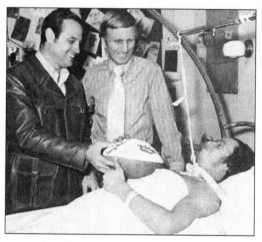

and propped up in a wheelchair, Gerry received the Outstanding Player Award at the banquet of the Brooklyn Club, a division of The Washington Touchdown Club. From the hospital bed, Gerry coordinated with the Alexandria Jaycee's a "Walk for Mankind." Gerry gathered students, adults, and company executives to donate. When Gerry was released from the hospital, he himself did 30 miles in his wheelchair.

Six months after the accident, Gerry returned to the football field – except this time he was to receive his diploma. At the graduation ceremony, Gerry wore a metal body brace and used crutches to half-drag, half-walk himself to the podium. There wasn't a dry eye there. Gerry was released from the hospital soon after graduation. Locally, Gerry was called by hospitals about depressed patients and he would come to visit and do a wheelie at the end of their bed.

When the patient was released he would go home with them and advise them how to do rehabilitation.

Gerry's mother heard him say, "I don't care if I'm paralyzed; God left me with my brain and I'm going to use it to help people less fortunate."

Gerry made speeches across the country to help handicapped individuals, and worked with the Alexandria city council to help establish and implement plans whereby handicapped persons could have access in and out of all the places we all take for granted. At Gerry's suggestion, the Alexandria Junior Chamber of Commerce started a "Ban the Barriers" project aimed at convincing store owners to eliminate architectural obstacles to wheelchairs.

Because of Gerry's great capacity to motivate, the incredulous works he performed for his fellow neighbor, and those across the United States, he was presented the "Presidents Award."

People throughout the United States have inquired about Gerry. Gerry went way beyond his football career that had been featured in "Remember the Titans." Even after his accident, Gerry never gave up and continued his successes until his death. On March 20, 1981, while on a business trip in Charlottesville, Va., Gerry was the victim of another horrifying auto accident. A drunk driver crossed the line and hit Gerry's car head on.

His adult years

Gerry is known for many different and wonderful things that include winning a Gold medal in the wheelchair Olympics in the "Shot-put" event, being chairman of "The Walk for Mankind" for many years, enrolled in Northern Virginia Community College, was active in the Alexandria Jaycees, and traveled everywhere, from coast to coast, speaking to clubs, schools, civic groups, and volunteering his time to dozens of organizations. He was living in his own apartment, driving his own car, and holding a full-time salesman's position.

Gerry had an underlying theme to all his civic work: to make the world a better place to live for those who were not so fortunate. "He was really something!" his mother Jean said. "The only difference between you all and Gerry is that you can stand up. He wasn't wasting away. He'd say, "Let's do something about life. It's not going to come to you."

Chapter 11

Logan Asks, "Are YOU the right girl for me?"

Dear potential girlfriend,

First of all, I realize that if you are reading this, and you are someone that I end up with; you probably don't need any convincing at all and already know everything I'm about to say. The right girlfriend for me won't need to read what I'm writing here in order for their mind to be changed in favor of me. But anyways, it needs to be said that I am just like every other single guy. I'm extremely interested in girls and desire a real, deep relationship with them (and one special one down the road, God willing). It's not like my condition alters my mind, maturity, and natural wants or needs. I want to be loved and to love just like the next guy. In fact, I'd say I'm one of the guys that wants and looks forward to that type of relationship more than some others do. I'm just really into and serious about that awesome part of life. I have no trouble saying that I go all out when it comes to it. That's how I am. Anyways, the only difference about me is my lack of physical ability due to Duchenne Muscular Dystrophy, which is something that I can do absolutely nothing about and shouldn't be something that cuts me short in the area of romance.

Unfortunately, because we're humans and sometimes we don't make complete sense; the fact is, it can and does put me somewhat behind in that department. I know because it has happened in the past. Several times I've had girls not take my interest in them very seriously because of my circumstance. They treat me like **the cute kid in a wheelchair,** and gush over my feelings for them like they would with a puppy. Maybe that description sounds a little bizarre, but I don't think I could come up with a better one. My close friends would agree with me because they experienced it right along with me, looking on. And though that was sort of a surprising and pretty painful issue for me earlier on in life, it kind of made sense in my mind; because if I were a girl I highly doubt I would be too excited to get with someone in a wheelchair. So, to be honest, I've gone through most of life expecting rejection from girls because I tried to see it through their eyes and experienced it quite a few times.

For a period of time, that negative leaning thinking was somewhat harmful to me because I never thought I would find someone. Thankfully, I know that's not true, because a few girls that **do get it** have popped up in my life here and there. I trust God that he will provide someone that's perfect for me at the right time. I also must admit that, occasionally in my situation's proneness for shallow treatment, I've fallen into the trap of shallowness in the past where I felt like I **had** to end up with one of the most attractive and well desired girls in order to prove that I was just like every other guy and could end up with the best. When I had that mentality, I would find myself being selfish in the midst of a situation where I can't afford that same sort of selfishness from the other end.

Through all of this and in the understanding I've developed, God has provided me with plenty of wisdom on what it means to **truly love** someone and also what it means to **truly be loved** by someone. I know that you, the right girl for me, won't handle my interest for you in the wrong way. I also know that when I find you I won't make the same mistakes in my mentality and will do so unselfishly. I look forward to and pray for our relationship to come every day as I wait for the Lord to bring us together.

With Love,
Logan

Chapter 12

School Days, Friendships, and Memories

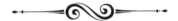

A h, those days at school when the childhood caterpillars grew into pupae, and then from the cocoon, butterflies broke free and took flight. From the first levels of instruction through high school, students go through a gauntlet of educational, emotional, physiological, romantic, and social experiences that molds them and shapes them for years to come. Things *don't have to be difficult*, but they sure can be.

- Teachers can be just out of college, or seasoned educators ready for retirement.
- The habits of teachers and administrators are as varied as in any industry anywhere. Some young teachers can act old, and some older teachers can act young-at-heart.
- Some students have solid home lives and good foundational role models in the home. Some students are exposed to parental dysfunction with screaming matches between the spouses which can cause high stress levels in the kids.
- Sibling interaction and rivalries can create a toxic environment that can increase parental stresses, and put students in a mindset not conducive to learning.
- Some students come from single-parent led homes. A child needs both a father and a mother figure to balance the

learning experience at home. It's tough enough with both parents; with a single parent, it really gets tough.
- Some students are near the poverty level. Some live where crime may be high.
- Some schools are under-funded, or resources are directed away from schools that need that allocation.

With all these factors rolled into the educational years in school, and then toss in an illness, debilitating condition, dramatic corrective surgeries, or other handicap, the trials can seem insurmountable. Logan Shannon faced these challenges very early in his education. So why does Logan have the optimism that he has when everything is factored in to his experience? What has made the difference in how Logan is where so many people have come 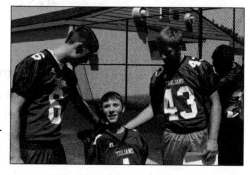 forward to contribute with letters in this book? Didn't he ever have disagreements with his sister or brothers while they were trying to get ready for school? Was each day always rosy in the Shannon garden of living when Logan needed so much assistance in getting all set with his homework, book bag, winter coat, and the participation in after school activities? What makes Logan tick? I wanted to know!

We are really beginning to see something unique with this young man. His effect on people extends far beyond just being a mutual classmate at school.

The head football coach for his high school, the Glen Este Trojans decided to honor Logan onto the football team his senior year by awarding him the jersey with #1 on it. How can a young man have that effect on people? Logan's younger brother was on the team, but it wasn't just that aspect which guided decisions by so many people.

How many people in a wheelchair would appreciate being decorated in a chariot and horses for the school mascot? Logan did.

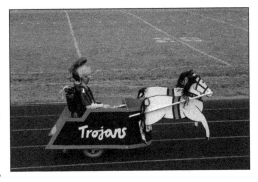

It took a lot of work by his friends and getting approval from coaching staff, but Logan easily was granted the job and won the hearts of hundreds of the students, parents, grandparents, and visitors to Glen Este High School Football games. I'm sure even visiting teams were known to inquire about this young man in the wheelchair as the mascot for the school. What do you think they were thinking?

Would it be possible that so many would embrace THIS student this way? Did this mean he was embraced by every student and every teacher in the whole school? I don't think there is that assumption at all.

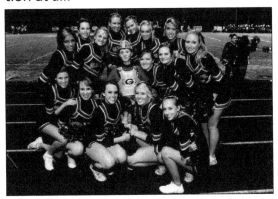

But imagine being welcomed by the cheerleaders at the home games through the "tunnel"! Logan Shannon was in that wheelchair for all four years of high school, and the mascot for three years. This was an honor, and he carried the responsibility with class, dignity, professionalism, energy, proficiency, and integrity.

There was always room for Logan when picture taking was going on. Why? Because he was appreciated. He focused on so many positive things, and didn't dwell on things that didn't matter.

Do you think he was treated this way just because he was in a wheelchair? Or would you consider they felt that way about **_Logan because of who he is?_**

Logan understood the complexity of his situation. He thought to tell his classmates a little about how he felt maturing alongside them. The thing that we can read from Logan's letter is that it could be told by anyone to their

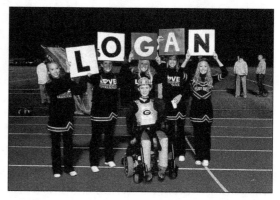

own group situation. Some may have a similar illness or condition that confines them to a mobile transportation device, so imagine you can take these and use them for your specific case. Read how Logan felt about this experience....

Dear school classmates,

I enjoyed getting to know the many of you over the years! I also really appreciate how all of you handled the unique situation of growing up with someone who deals with Duchenne Muscular Dystrophy like me. When I think about it, we were privileged with a pretty cool learning experience to go through together where you guys were able to learn how to interact with someone physically disabled and I was able to learn what different initial reactions I may come across with different people.

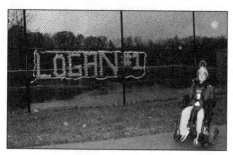

As ridiculous as it sounds, I definitely went through a phase of time where I felt like I needed to basically prove to the kids that I dealt with on a regular basis that I was (and am) just like everyone else.

"As ridiculous as it sounds, I definitely went through a phase of time where I felt like I needed to basically prove to the kids that I dealt with on a regular basis that I was (and am) just like everyone else.."

Over time, you guys revealed to me that I really had little, if any, proving of myself to do. From what I saw (and still see), you all knew I was just as normal as the rest of you and at some point, all of you came to treating me this way as well. I will say that some of you might've grasped this understanding a little later than others, but I really get that and have no issue with anyone who fits into that category.

It's a situation that most young people don't face and I don't think you guys could have handled it any better. By the way, you handled it better in our process of maturing than most full-grown adults do.

Those who I have known since elementary school at Clough Pike had a real advantage in knowing how to handle it because they knew me even before muscular dystrophy reached the obvious severity of being wheelchair bound. I am especially grateful for those of you who fit into that time frame because you really did a great job of showing the rest of our classmates, through middle and high school, how ordinary, humanly speaking, I am; and how they could interact with me the same way they interact with everyone else. You did a wonderful job at **taking charge and leading by example** in this aspect. That may not seem like much, or even

"It's a situation that most young people don't face and I don't think you guys could have handled it any better. By the way, you handled it better in our process than most full-grown adults do."

like you did anything at all, but believe me when I say it was big and meant a lot to me.

I am amazed at the number of close and lifelong friends I have made with so many of our class. I truly value all the friendships that were developed with each and every one of you over the years. I hope these words are an encouragement and blessing to all of you! It is my desire that you can look back on how we interacted with each other and in that reflection understand the significance of everything I've written here. God bless you and your families in whatever you are doing now and will do in the future!

Sincerely,
Logan Shannon

Now let's hear from Vicki Henshey, one of Logan's teachers as she remembers Logan from the 2nd grade:

Dear Logan,

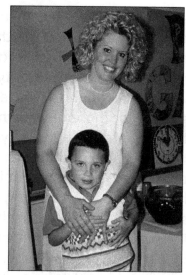

Many years ago, when you walked into my 2nd grade classroom, I could have never imagined the impact you would have on my life. You were just another bright-eyed seven-year-old who may have been a bit more wobbly, and perhaps a bit smaller than the other boys, but you had more spunk and had a greater passion for learning than the others. At that time, I was not aware that on that very day, I not only became your teacher, I became your admirer.

My initial memory of you as a second grader takes me to the hallway, outside of our classroom that took us towards the cafeteria and the restrooms. I so vividly see you and twenty-something of your fellow classmates walking in a single-file line behind me, like little ducklings following their momma. As the leader of the line, I would walk backwards, always being on the lookout for you. Your little muscles were beginning to fail you a bit, and although you were not yet wheel-chair bound, you would often gently collapse into a little heap as you walked. My job, as we walked down that hallway, was for you to know that I would be there to scoop you up, so you could continue down the hall with your friends. This was just what we did and no one thought much about it. Your classmates knew your diagnosis and although they were empathetic, they treated you no different, except that they may have loved you a little more than their other friends.

During that 2nd grade year, the class became pen pals with another classroom of students. My son Colten was your pen pal. Yes, I hand-picked him to correspond with you because I wanted him to know you, and also feel your spirit. The two of you became friends, although it was a bit awkward since the both of you attended

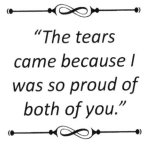

"The tears came because I was so proud of both of you."

different elementary schools and were not at all talkative at that time of your lives. But, I remember how excited he was when he found out you were coming to his magician-themed birthday party that year, and ten years later, to his graduation party. As the two of you sang together in a high school choir concert and spoke as top students of your graduating class….. you as

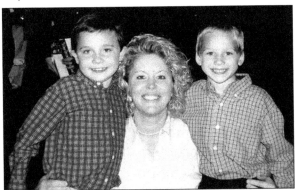

Valedictorian of Glen Este and he as Salutatorian of Amelia, I cried. The tears came because I was so proud of both of you. How your life journeys seemed parallel in so many ways, yet such polar opposites.

Our lives are better for knowing you. I know God placed you in my life for a multitude of reasons, but I like to think it was just to be one of the many who love you and who are inspired by you. You are a precious gift, Logan.

Blessings,

Mrs. Henshey (then a 2nd grade teacher at Clough Pike Elementary School)

The picture on the previous page shows another boy with Mrs. Henshey who was not the pen pal mentioned, but Logan's younger brother, Devon (who started at the same elementary school one grade year behind Logan).

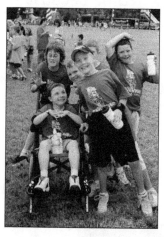

The interesting thing is that Logan was accepted by classmates from even the earliest times in elementary school. He was involved in plays, sports, outdoor activities, and group play time as the progression of Duchenne Muscular Dystrophy advanced. In fact, Logan was often in the middle of all kinds of fun because he **viewed himself** as part of the group that **viewed him** as just one of them!

He was in a wheelchair? So what! Just "Fuggettaboutit!!"

Field trips? No problem. Theme events like the 5th grade luau event? No problem. What about the School Walkathon? No problem. What about one getting it going on

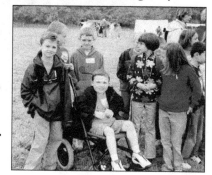

the dance floor? No problem. What about just messing around during school recess? No problem.

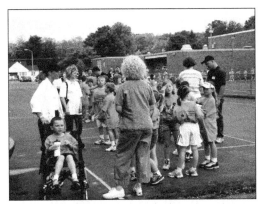

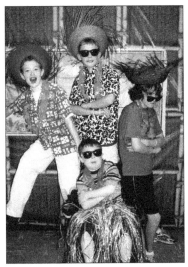

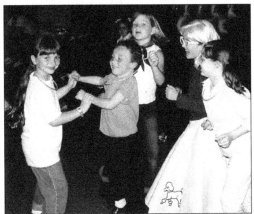

Logan also chose to write a letter to the Glen Este High School Principal – Mr. John Speiser:

Dear Mr. Spieser,

I want to thank you for the period of time you spent as my principal at Glen Este High School. I really appreciated the way that you ran things. You were very personable, patient, and kind to your students. Along with this friendly demeanor, it was very clear to me that

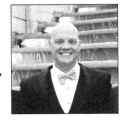

you would do whatever it took to stand up for what is right. You made it obviously known what you believe to be right, and at the same time, worked with students rather than forcing them into a certain mold of following the rules. I always respected you for going about everything in that way. You seem to really get how this world operates and understand that everyone's life takes a completely different path to get where God means for them to be.

To be honest, I do consider you to be somewhat of a friend after all of my experiences around you. You are one of those rare people that I come across that immediately, upon initial interaction, treats me just like everyone else and pays basically no attention to my differences due to muscular dystrophy. With most people it takes a little bit of time before they understand there really is nothing different about me.

And that simply wasn't the case with you. For some reason I always sensed that you knew I was capable of doing great things amidst my physical disabilities. I don't know if it was the way you watched me, how you were always willing to help me, or simply the tone of the conversations we had together. It was probably a little bit of all of those. This became especially evident to me during my senior year.

During that time, I could tell you really thought highly of me and hope you could tell the same from me. You supported me all the way through everything on the way to being one of our valedictorians, and were just as excited as I was about what the future holds for me. So, it came as no surprise to me when you allowed me to share the gospel and what my relationship with Jesus means to me for my graduation speech. Thank you so much for approving such a speech to be given, because I know you easily could have knocked it down in concern for the politically correct crowd found in our society. You have no idea how much I appreciate it! That closing moment of my senior year was really the pinnacle of my entire high school career. Everything I do is built upon the message of Jesus Christ, so for me to get that message out there means everything to me. And, in part, because of you I was able to do that in front of my peers and thousands of others. It was a pretty amazing and powerful end to my time, and your time as well, at Glen Este High School! Once again, I want to thank you for all that you did for me during that time. I hope that all is well with you and your family! I'm praying for you and God bless you at your new job as principal at Clark Montessori!

Sincerely,
Logan Shannon

And that same principal, John Spieser wrote a letter; and told Logan how he felt about him:

Dear Logan,

I have memories. Lots of memories. Who do I remember, especially from school? All students have a place in there. Some occupy more space than others. Some are imbedded deeper than others. But all have importance. Does it mean that if they occupy more space that it means I

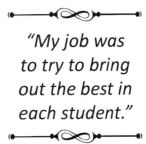

"My job was to try to bring out the best in each student."

liked them better? No. Does it mean if you've made a greater impact on me or the school, that I liked you better? No. My job was to try to bring out the best in each student. And I wanted that. I didn't want any student to achieve or attain something that wasn't them. And each student was different and would hang out with friends that complimented the group or disrupted the group. Some were brash. Some preferred to be in the

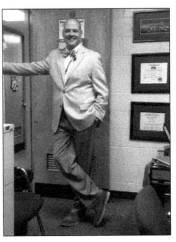

background. Some made great leaders and some great followers. Some reached for superior grades. Some reached for superior popularity. Some reached for sports excellence. Some reached for the quiet acceptance that they would simply strive for completion of school. Some struggled with incredible hardship in family situations, financial capacity, or emotional acceptance in social circles. But each and every student had equal weight with me.

Logan Shannon stood out in a very unique way. Logan was a sophomore and wheelchair bound when I started as principal. I continued as principal through his senior year, and moved to another school in the Cincinnati area after the 2012 – 2013 school year. So it was hard to miss Logan, because there was always a potential that his wheelchair would find its way into your shins if you got out of line...... (wink)

One thing I thought about that Logan helped me with personally, was he made me more aware of how others perceive him. My wife and I adopted a child from another country because of a heart-felt tugging that initiated the process. We occasionally get stares on because our child doesn't have the genetics to "match" us, and I can tell people try to figure it out (as if it needed to be figured out). Logan has noticed out of the corner of his eye that people may have been staring, I'm sure. The way Logan progressed through the years while I was principal displayed maturity, grace, and accountability.

"Logan Shannon stood out in a very unique way. Logan was a sophomore and wheel chair bound when I started as principal."

I always liked the Glen Este school spirit and I liked to dress the part in school colors, purple and white, especially on those big game days!

Some of my best memories in the sports aspect was the excitement of football games and the school pride we had. Some of Logan's friends even came up with a contraption that fit over his wheelchair that looked like the Trojans mascot chariot, complete with horses!

That's the way his friends were. There was a special type of resurgence of camaraderie between Logan and his friends. It was great to see. There was fooling around as if he wasn't even in a wheelchair. And Logan's friends were fine students, a respectable core group.

1) I can't remember any of his group in detention.
2) They followed the rules and had me pre-approve "senior pranks" that they intended to do. They were not destructive, always in good fun.
3) They expressed great school spirit.

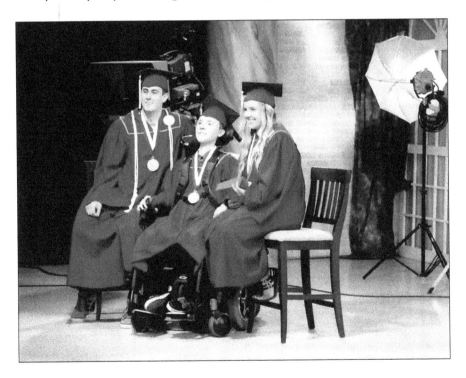

Some may have thought that the valedictorian address that Logan gave was inappropriate. But I didn't think so.

His address was a spiritual challenge to all the graduates and their families and friends. He spoke of his faith (in Jesus Christ), and explained how that worked. He spoke of how his faith sustained him in many rough moments and situations. I never gave it a thought about him sharing his faith because it was genuine and it was **who** Logan was. He spoke from the heart and with complete sincerity. I was not going to deny him from telling that. By the way, all feedback from those in attendance was **totally** positive with **no** negatives.

In closing, I wanted to say these things about Logan from my personal experience:

1) I have no real words of encouragement for Logan. He is the one who is the inspiration for the rest of **us**. He encourages us by his words and actions.

2) There is such a gracious spirit about him that's contagious. His positive outlook shines.

3) Whenever Logan entered a room, the atmosphere seemed to change. It was really something to witness.

4) He has an inner strength and courage that's hard to miss. He is in quite a situation being confined to that wheelchair, yet exudes a confidence that inspires.

5) Too many of us take so many things for granted. He was able to reach a high level of achievement, keep an awesome core group of friends, maintain civility with administration and student groups, and still present himself as just one of the guys. Despite his obvious physical limitation, Logan was a tremendous asset to our school.

Logan, take care, my friend.
All the best,

John Spieser, Glen Este High School Principal 2010 – 2013

Speaking of principals, Steve Brokamp was Logan's principal at Clough Pike Elementary School and wrote:

Dear Logan,

Many people come into our lives, and that population seems to increase, exponentially, as the years pass and our acquaintances expand their families. Acquaintances become friends, friends become family, and families are blessed with children. Such was the case when we made the life altering decision to build a home in a new section of our neighborhood, two doors down from your parents.

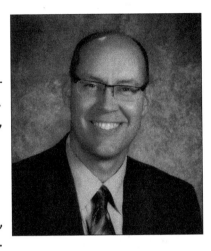

At that time, you were a plan in the making. Your parents were preparing for you before you ever came into this world. Of course, you know the rest of the story, or at least the story that has been written up until now. Perhaps, however, you are now learning a bit more about the intricate details of your own story web. There is a theory in mathematics and science called "chaos." Essentially, the theory recognizes that changes, no matter how small, can give rise to strikingly great consequences. It's like a domino effect on steroids. One event gives rise to a chain of events. Logan, you are that lead domino. You have touched so many lives in such positive ways. The beautiful thing to behold is that your web, your "chaos," and your "domino trail" continues forever and expands continuously. It is your legacy.

I have known for many years that you were perfectly placed on this Earth. Think about it. You have been given everything you need to live a life perfectly suited to your exceptionalism. Your parents are devout Christians, whose faith only grew stronger because of the blessings you, along with your siblings, provided. Their knowledge of physical therapy combined with their extraordinary patience, understanding, and peace, which comes only as a result of their faith, was further proof that you were perfectly placed. Your siblings are top scholars, strong Christians, and phenomenal people in every way. Your teachers have been top notch. Your friends, your teams, your neighborhood, your cul-de-sac, your church, and your organizations have been outstanding supports filled with wonderful people. I have been blessed to witness it all. As your neighbor, friend, coach, principal, and I dare say "member of your family," I have been witness to things about your development that, perhaps, no one else has.

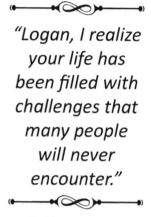

"Logan, I realize your life has been filled with challenges that many people will never encounter."

Logan, I realize your life has been filled with challenges that many people will never encounter. I realized when you were small that there were forces at work placing you on a different path. I remember the struggles you had taking your first steps, running, swinging a bat, getting down the hallways at school, functioning as a student in a school filled with "ordinary kids." All the while, at least initially, other kids were curious and unsure of how to talk with you, how to include you, how to laugh with you and play with you. To make matters more difficult, you learned that not only was your physical condition challenging, but it would likely become more difficult very soon. These changes came at the same moment when your peers would become physically stronger, faster, and more coordinated. How you have handled all of these challenges has been nothing short of inspirational. Logan, through your example you have inspired me to be better. I strive, daily, to be a person who faces challenges with grace, compassion, and kindness. You are one of a few extraordinary examples I think about when I cope with my own challenges. I know you would agree, through our adversity, we become stronger, better, and more faith-filled, if we allow it.

Logan, you have made me a better friend by realizing the importance of reaching out and including others. In fact, unlikely friendships are the most precious of all, because differences and obstacles are tossed aside, exposing the true soul of a person. You have made me a better neighbor by being blessed with the opportunity to associate with you on a daily basis. (I miss those daily opportunities, by the way.)

You have made me a better coach. Because your strength now prevented you from holding the bat up very long, I became the best at placing balls perfectly over the plate, exactly where I knew your bat would fall? (smile). Do you remember your teammates waiting inside the base-ball field backstop for the opportunity to run **for** you when your bat made contact with the ball? Do you remember your ele-mentary school principal (me)? He was perfectly placed to learn from you and see you through. Do you remember the countless hours that we played together in the cul-de-sac? How many times do you remember adults and kids playing together, as one family, so long into the night that we pulled our grills to the end of the driveway on occasion just so we didn't have to stop playing while we made dinner? Then, like any functional family, we prayed and ate together.

"Do you remember your teammates waiting inside the baseball field backstop for the opportunity to run for you when your bat made contact with the ball? "

I hope by now you realize what has been going on. You are, in fact, exceptional and you make those around you exceptional. That is the power of extraordinary people. If you were ordinary, much of what I described above would not have happened. What "chaos" would have transpired had you not tipped the correct dominoes?

I can assure you, you are exceptional; not only because you are different, but because you have embraced your uniqueness and tailored your path to fit your unique promise and hope. And here is the message that resonates with me more than any other... **Your exceptionalism is your gift.** Your weakness (if you can call it that) is your strength. It is what compels you, motivates you, gets you noticed, and makes you stand out. It has taught you patience, persistence, and even inner peace. It has not come without price, but you have handled yourself amazingly well, and that is exactly why I am so proud to know you. I know what I am about to say seems a little dramatic, but it is true... You have faced and overcome fears that would crush ordinary men, even extraordinary men.

Logan, you have made everyone around you better. That is the true measure of a leader. Your parents, though faithful, would not be the same, faith-filled Christians they are today if it were not for you and your siblings. Together, you have motivated them and given them a higher purpose. Your siblings have done amazing things for you and with you, but that relationship has been reciprocal. They have been forever strengthened through their relationship with you. And what about my family? Miss Andi, Christoper (Oey), Jason, Jaxie, and I love you more than you may ever know. Thank you for being our friend, classmate, teammate, lunch buddy, student, neighbor, inspiration, but mostly thank you for being YOU! No one else could ever hope to do that better! Continue the good work!

"Logan, you have made everyone around you better. That is the true measure of a leader."

God bless you, and again, we love you

Steve Brokamp; friend, neighbor, principal, coach, and admirer.

Chapter 13

Four Friends Share Their Letters

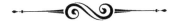

B rad Young, Brian Wirthlin, Jo Ferro, and Joey Speigel all know Logan, and offer their heart-felt affection for their friend!

Brad Young has known Logan since middle school, and their friendship continues to this day. He shares the initial encounter with Logan on an opposing little league baseball team. He goes on to share what it was like to hear Logan whizzing around the school hallways along with the impact Logan's faith has made on him.

Brian Wirthlin made his way into Logan's core of friends in 7th grade and still remains in Logan's close circle. He, too, experienced his first encounter at the ball field, and speaks of his gradual pursuit of becoming one of Logan's comrades. In typical Brian fashion, he mentions some of the inner circle's more crazy shenanigans.

Jo Ferro has known Logan for years through mutual friends. They became close during Logan's junior year and her sophomore year as, shall we say, she was one of the first girls to see him for who he really is. Their friendship will always be important to Logan. She speaks of Logan's impact in her walk with Christ.

Joey Speigel has been close with Logan since their earliest elementary school years. Like Brad and Brian, he remembers being profoundly affected by watching Logan playing baseball.

He shares how they bonded through their mutual love of sports and faith in God. He recounts the progression of their friendship over the years.

First, Brad Young:

Dear Logan,

When everything on your body worked, there were baseball games to be played! You may not remember the first time we met, but I do. We were both super young and played baseball at the Tealtown Baseball League complex, you for the Rangers and I for the Eagles. This was before you had your wheelchair and you were always 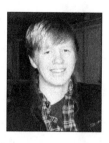 a good sport and loved the game. I don't know why that old memory has always stuck with me, but playing against you in that baseball game as kids, has just always been a memory of mine, and a good one at that. I didn't know it then, but it sowed the seeds of friendship that would grow and grow......

We first became friends in middle school. Back then, it seemed we'd just sit in class, go to lunch, and go back and sit in class again. This seemed to go on and on and on. It felt like such a boring time looking back on it now, but somehow I saw you as always so positive at school. It was always a good day when I saw you chilling and yacking it up at the end of one of the lunch tables.

There you were; joking around and ***living life*** at a place that isn't always the happiest place on earth, and ***living that life*** in a chair-shaped machine that many think is not the happiest thing to be in. And I wasn't the only one at the school who noticed, either. Sometimes we HEARD you before we SAW you! And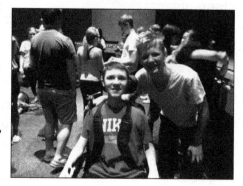

it wasn't from your voice, either. I think some of my favorite memories (and I don't know if we ever told you this) was when we could always tell when you were going down the hall while we were in class. We could hear the faint whirring of your motorized wheelchair as you made your way echoing down the hallway. It got louder and louder and louder, and we all seemed to drift

from what the teachers were saying to the empty doorway opening. Then WHOOOSHHH; you would fly by the doorway opening at full speed on your wheelchair and I couldn't help but chuckle every time you went by. Sometimes, even teachers would notice. Others would laugh, too. It was just like some big anticipation you knew was coming by the sound getting louder and louder, and then when you flew by, we cracked up. And then the sound faded away. And it was funny just because you would 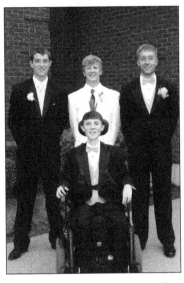 be completely oblivious to what it sounded like to us *inside* the classroom. It was funny to so many other students, too.

There are always more funny stories that we shared, but I believe the first thing I will always think of when I hear the name Logan Shannon is your faith in Jesus Christ. I could never put my finger on it, but there was something special about the way you loved God and loved people as a response to God's love. It was always inspiring to *my* faith to say the least. And you always seemed to know the right thing to say. No matter the question, no matter the circumstance; you were just knowledgeable and shared your wisdom when it came to questions about Jesus and living out a Christian life. I promise you I wasn't the only one seeing this either! The entire high school, faculty and students, knew exactly who you were and what you were about, and you were about spreading God's love to all. It was truly amazing back then, and is still to this day!

And even at this point in time, I know I can always turn to you for anything, whether it's a personal ride to my car on the platform on the back of your wheelchair or a question regarding the

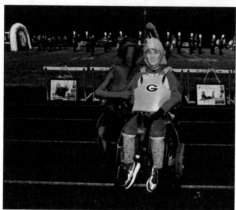

deepest of theology. In any of those cases, I know you will always "point" me in the right direction. You are one of my best friends, an inspirational man of Christ, and the way you live your life is living proof that there is a God, he is Almighty, and he loves each and every one of us. And any person would be able to sense that if they ever met you. I love you, man. You're an amazing friend!

Your brother in Christ,
Brad Young

Now from Brian Wirthlin:

Logan,

We were Avengers!! Fighting crime and rescuing the innocent! Remember? Don't shake your head. I KNOW you remember! We should have won that costume contest at the midnight movie premiere! All of the kids HAD to get a picture with the Avengers, led by famous

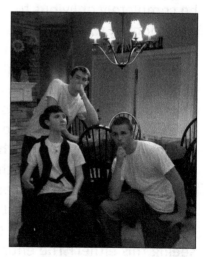

Logan "Nick Fury" Shannon, complete with the eye patch! The

night was ours, and we were invincible! Of course, until we had to wake up for school at 7 o'clock the next morning...

So when did our friendship start? Picture day for little league baseball was the first time I saw you, so we must have been in first or second grade at the time. The sun was dodging from behind clouds off and on, but it was a pretty nice day. Your teammates were being coached into position by the adults for the group photo, and it seemed at one point that they were all looking towards you as you slowly walked over to join them. In fact, many others watched you, too. After several uncertain steps, you joined the team. Then everyone smiled for the camera 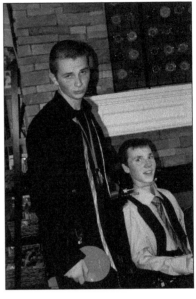 and the small crowd of parents and coaches smiled back. I doubt you remember me being there. It seemed like an insignificant moment at the time, but that moment in time is burned into my memory. I kept seeing you from time to time at the ball fields, and at school.

But I actually met you for the first time when we were in seventh grade. This is another time burned into my memory. I was just an awkward kid with a "not so cool" haircut sitting at the end of your lunch table. I definitely did not belong on the "cool side" with you guys. Your end of the table always seemed much more appealing to me. Why? I don't know exactly, but probably because I knew in my heart that you were one of my soon-to-be best friends. You were always smiling. Smiling! Here you were in a wheelchair, and I watched a group of guys laughing and not only ***living life***, but ***doing life*** together. You didn't seem to fit the mold of feeling sorry for yourself. You were too busy being you to be concerned. I knew I wanted ***that*** type of community, and I wanted whatever gave you the joy that I saw in you. I didn't know how I was going to become your friend, and I kind of talked to myself about how to do it. So I settled on first just kind of being around you. Then, to be recognized by you, then to participate with you. After that, I felt we'd become friends.

Eventually in high school, I did become a part of this inner circle, quickly realizing that none of us were cool by any means. Our collective failed attempts at interacting with the ladies proved that. Who cares anyway? We always had fun and created plenty of memories. Like the time that Trevor threw that paper airplane, and it ended up hitting you in the face? We all cracked up when that happened. Okay, maybe we thought it was funnier than you did..... How about special and memorable stuff? Like football 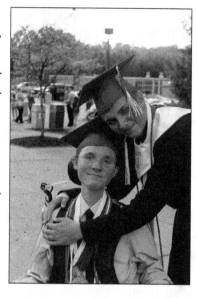 games every Friday night, where you became the best mascot Glen Este High School had ever seen? That chariot contraption fitted over your wheelchair was one of the best ideas! And then we went over the edge when we were the hottest male cheerleaders at the powder puff games? Think that's all? Nah....... You know I HAVE to mention the time that you let one rip during our physics exam. The whole room lost control, and I'm not sure how Boyle's Law was involved in that "great escape"! Plus, it was so incredible that you allowed everyone to blame it on Joey Speigel. Good luck ever living that acoustic interruption down.

But Logan, on a serious note; I want to share some deep thoughts with you. Even after holding many doors and getting my toes run over by your wheelchair countless times, you have become one of my best friends. I know I can always stop by the Shannon household whenever I am hungry or just need a place

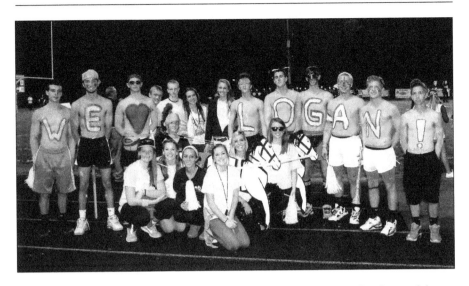

to go. You have shown me so much about your faith and how Jesus is working through you, which only helps my faith grow stronger. Your ministry is not only through your words, but also in *the example* you set with your life. You continuously show me what it looks like to follow God wherever He leads, and how to give Him complete control. You have taught me how to deal with life's obstacles by keeping faith in God's greater plans. When most of us become isolated and feel defeated in our struggles, you always run to Jesus first.

You have demonstrated how to be transparent, truthful, and authentic with your friends and family. And you also know how to rely on the power of community and prayer.

I realize that your body is getting weaker and weaker. Despite that, you are the strongest man I know, because your strength comes from the One that is bigger than any obstacle we can face. In your graduation speech, you summed it up with, "*He* is the source of my strength, *He* is the strength of my life". Even if you don't realize it, you have taught me this time and time again. I cannot put into words how much of a blessing your friendship has been to me.

I am convinced that when I first saw you fifteen years ago, God was showing me that our stories would intersect at some day in the future. I have watched you do many courageous and incredible things with the short time that we have been here on this planet. But I know that it is not over, and that God is still showing us new stuff. The plans He has in store for you are bigger than anything you or I could possibly imagine, and I can't wait to see where they take you.

Love you buddy!
Brian Wirthlin

Then Ms. Jo Ferro contributes:

Dear Logan,

How many girls can say they have been serenaded? Not many.....

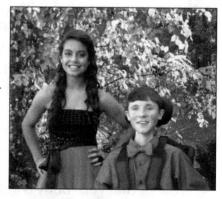

This is just one reason why I'll never forget you. I'll never forget how fast we became friends and how close we came to be. You were a great listener and helped me put some things in perspective when I was going through a stressful year at school. However, what I was going through at school was nothing compared to what you go through every day.

Nonetheless you treated me as though my thoughts and worries were valid and never belittled me or made me feel petty though sometimes I probably deserved it.

I'll never forget the 16th birthday gift you gave me, which included 16 gifts (to make up for all the birthdays you missed). Each of the 16 items were something I had told you that I wanted at one point in time; from pudding, to a New England Patriots football jersey, you remembered it all.

I'll never forget your great sense of humor and how you were able to laugh at yourself and politely laugh at other people too. The one thing that I will **always remember** is the reason why you were able to be so caring, and to have such a wonderful sense of humor and to love unconditionally: your faith in Jesus Christ. In everything you did and said, you were intentional to display your faith and your reliance on the Lord. I truly believe that your faith in God is the only thing that enables you to live the passionate and motivated life that you live.

I want you to know that you have had a profound impact on my life and have made me want to be a better servant of Christ. I wish that I and everyone else were more like you.

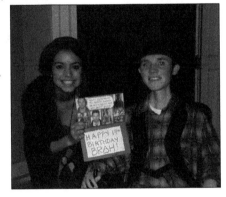

Thank you for being a great friend to me, one that I don't deserve. Praise God for people like Logan Shannon.

In Christian Love,
Jo Ferro

Then to close this chapter, Joey Speigel submits his letter:

Logan,

I still remember the first time I ever saw Logan. At our home town baseball field my family and I were just arriving for my tee ball game. As we approached our field there was a game still going on, that game happened to be Logan's. The next player came to bat and I thought it would be just like all the rest. However, this at bat was different, the crowd got on their feet and began to cheer. As the boy swung and hit the ball, he ran to first, the crowd went wild! I didn't know what the big deal was, to me it was just another routine little hit for a base hit. It wasn't until after the game that I found out that boy had Duchenne Muscular Dystrophy, and that boy who swung that bat was Logan Shannon.

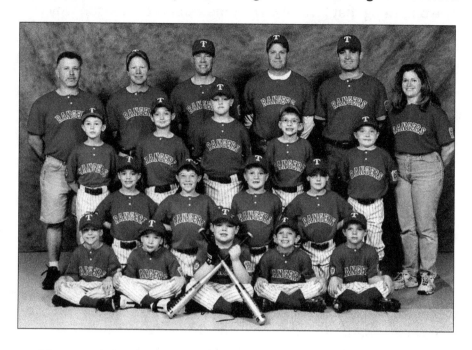

The ensuing school year is when I really got to meet Logan, we were both starting first grade at Clough Pike Elementary. We had a couple interactions but it wasn't until the 4th or 5th grade that Logan and I really became good friends. In fact, Logan and I joke about not actually liking each other early on because we both were so competitive. But when we really got to know each other we began to bond on our love for sports and strong faith in God.

Then through middle school, Logan and I were all interested in the same things, which worked out great. I was able to help him with his needs in class and at the same time I got to be in all the same classes with my best friend, which was just a bonus for us!

What was so great about our friendship was that, that's exactly what it was. Logan never demanded or expected me to do things for him and I never felt like I HAD to do things for him or only helped him because I was "supposed" to. We just did it, he was my friend, and I was his. We always looked at it as that's just what friends do. The thing with Logan was he was always so patient with me and our other friends when helping him. His patience is a trait, I myself wish I had. The amount of strength Logan has is unreal. Due to his condition, I'm not talking about physical strength but mental strength. Logan never complained about his condition.

In school, or wherever, he wanted to be treated equal and went about his day as if he didn't have his disease at all. What was most notable was that I knew, my friends knew, and anyone who knew Logan knew where his strength came from. That strength **was** and *is* Jesus Christ, our Savior.

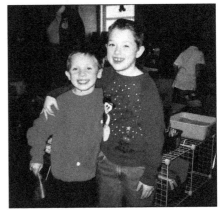

Unfortunately, because of Logan's condition, he was never able to play sports, but that never stopped him from being a sports fanatic. I played both football and basketball through high school and there are very few games that I remember looking over to that sideline and not seeing Logan cheering us on. Senior year was the most memorable year for me with Logan. That year for football, Logan became a part of the team.

He was our mascot and our honorary number one fan. My friends and I made Logan a chariot that attached to his wheel chair. This really vamped up his "mascoting" abilities, even though he was already the best mascot in the Nation!

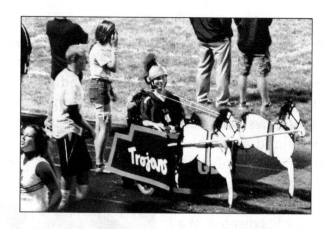

Senior year we had the "Coach To Cure MD" game against Turpin. Even though we lost the game it was one of the most amazing nights of my life. I got to go out and play football for my best friend, all in bringing awareness to help find a cure for Logan.

The second half of senior year took a little bit of a rough turn for me. I went down some roads that I wish I hadn't and got into a little bit of trouble. I believe a lot of this happened because I only had one class with Logan that year. I lost my strong rock that kept me straight for so long. Now Logan and I were still close but 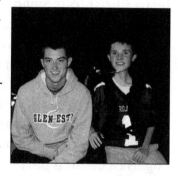 those few months were rough. I know Logan prayed very strongly for me and, after hitting rock bottom, I was able to bounce back and Logan was right there to welcome me with open arms. Senior year ended great for the both of us and graduating was a proud moment for us. But the highlight of senior year was Logan's Valedictorian speech. At our graduation ceremony, Logan gave a speech that I will never forget, he spoke in front of thousands and strictly gave praise to God for getting him this far and giving him the abilities that he has. His speech was so moving, it brought tears to my eyes. As much

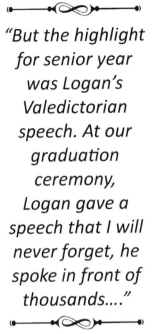

"But the highlight for senior year was Logan's Valedictorian speech. At our graduation ceremony, Logan gave a speech that I will never forget, he spoke in front of thousands…."

as I don't like talking about it, Logan very well could have not made it to graduation day. But God gave him the strength to not only graduate but to be our class Valedictorian!! Praise God for that!

When I graduated, I had a scholarship to go play football in Indiana. I was going to go to school to be a teacher and looking forward to starting my future. However, God had different plans for me. Some things happened between my parents and I which left me with a huge decision on what to do about college. I spoke with my friends and family on what to do, but was still lost. However, one day while working out for football I felt God's presence. All of a sudden, I started to think about Logan, and how we have always been together and now I might possibly be leaving him. Also, I realized all of Logan's and my friends were going away to college as well. I knew I needed to stay home and be here with him. Then all the years of helping Logan and being his aide came to mind. God then gave me the decision. I was to stay at home and go to our community college and go for nursing. Never before had I thought of this, but I knew God's hand was upon it. Not too long after that, I decided to stay home and knew it was a great decision. Logan and I began spending a lot of time together. I was blessed enough to be trusted by his parents that I was able to drive Logan around in his family van. It allowed for me and Logan to do so many more things together.

Logan decided to take a year off from school. But as I started my freshman year of college, Logan and I thought it'd be a great idea to start our own Bible study for our local friends still in town. This was just the start for Logan and his journey with Christ.

Logan decided not to go to school and just focus on his Faith, and what a difference it made.

Logan soon solely began to run the Bible studies as my schooling became very overwhelming. However, Logan embraced it and shortly those once a week bible studies became the high-light of my week.

Now being three years out of high school, Logan's faith has gone beyond measure. The love he has for God is astounding. The knowledge that he possesses about God amazes me every time we speak about our Faith. His will to live and live for Christ is what helps me to be a better Christian and overall better person. Since the very first day I met Logan I knew God put him on this Earth to change it, and this book is just the start.

Joey Spiegel

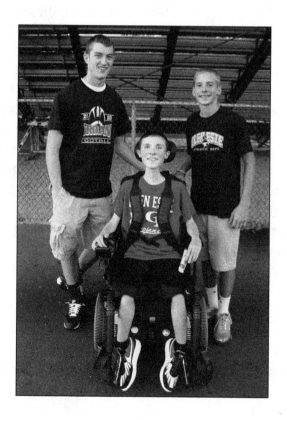

Chapter 14

Logan's Family - They All Share Their Hearts

To Mom (Tyra) and from Mom, to Dad (Michael) and from Dad, to Logan's older sister (Sydney) and hers to Logan, to Logan's next younger brother (Devon) and his to Logan, and to Logan's youngest brother (Corey), and his to Logan.

Dear Mom,

It is obviously a far different experience having a son with Duchenne Muscular Dystrophy than it is having an "ordinary" child like Sydney, Devon, and Corey (if you can even call them that)! There's simply just a lot more things I have needed and still need assistance with. And you know that more than anyone, Mom! There actually is a lot more I need than anyone would think just looking at the surface, because of that we often lovingly declare that most people just don't get it! We have been brought through the wringer, and even brought each other through the wringer, time and time again because of the complex difficulty of our situation.

Being honest, many times that gets frustrating and even overwhelming to both of us! And we've dealt with that since early on, because none of this is easy! Through it all, we have learned a ton about each other and it has become pretty easy for us to be transparent and real with each other in every circumstance. So it has always been easier for me to come to you than anyone else with most of my needs. So in terms of mother-son relationships, we are extremely close. I am so thankful for that! That's been one of the hidden blessings of this ongoing trial, because without it there's no way we would have as much real love and understanding for each other as we do! *You have been tested* as a mother to come to a place of complete willingness to drop everything to come to the aid of your child and *I have been tested* to accept that even in my dependence I will not and cannot be the obvious, immediate priority all the time. You and I can both agree that, though it's hard to see sometimes, the benefit and growth from what we face far outweigh the pain and perceived cost of each situation.

You have been so patient with me! I admit that I am not always as sensitive to your needs as you are to mine. I've gone through phases where I've felt victimized by my circumstance and felt almost as though it's only fair for me to want 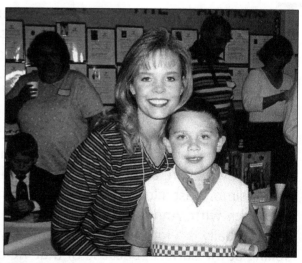 everything I need; and to get it right when I need it. Thank you for sticking with me through it all, especially when I definitely don't deserve it!

We've been growing as individuals and followers of Jesus with each other all along. There have been endless ups and downs that we've faced with each other, ups and downs that are completely different and more severe than any average ups and downs, I feel necessary to add. There is no doubt about how much we care for each other! That goes for the whole family really; we're the only ones who truly understand the hardships! As dividing as Muscular Dystrophy can be at times, it has been an overall unifying circumstance for our family because we're really going through it AS a family. And you have been the one to make sure of it! For that, you truly are amazing, Mom! Amidst all the difficulty and lessons, what I've really needed from you is just for you to be there to love me, hold me, and comfort me through all the rough days from any situation.

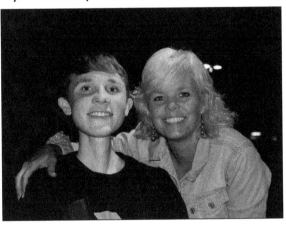

You have done just that and so, so, so much more! I'm in a position that is extremely vulnerable and it's easiest for me to be vulnerable with my mom. So in my vulnerability, I've been vulnerable with you. Other ones, like Tom Sulfaro (chapter 9) have a brother who is the closest. Those with DMD know their vulnerability, and need that someone who will always be there.

Mom, you've been there to listen to me and to hug me. A lot! I have absolutely needed it. We don't know all the reasons why, but we've been chosen to be in this position. Since we've been chosen, God has promised we will be able to handle it. You have been a perfect example of the fact that it's much harder and very nearly impossible for us to handle it on our own. And that we must rely on the Lord instead. Thank you for all that you mean to me and do for me!

Love, Your Son,
Logan

Now Mom's letter to her son, Logan:

My Dearest Logan,

Loving you has been one of my life's greatest joys. As the Lord saw fit to knit you in my womb and allow me the privilege of giving birth to a beautiful baby boy; you became our second born child following your big sister, but our first son. On January 25, 1995, after nearly delivering you in the elevator at the hospital because your Dad stopped at the light to search in the console to find a piece of gum, my journey of motherhood increased double fold.

Though I was longing to be a mommy of many children, I was also scared to death. I once again fell head over heels in love with another little being as the doctor placed you in my arms. As I held you, I knew life would never be the same again. Not only once, but twice, I had been given a good and perfect gift from my heavenly Father. Although it's impossible to see the future, I pondered the road ahead, trying to imagine what it might look like while holding on to the precious present moment.

I asked God a second time, "What will I do with this tiny being that is relying on me for life and growth?" And in a tender whisper, in the depths of my heart, He gave me the same answer.....Love him well, love him unconditionally and love him like I love you.

From day one you and I entered the classroom with Sydney. I was learning how to manage two babies 15 months apart in age while you and your sister were endlessly exploring new life. I treasured every season we walked through together. From all the bonding experiences of diaper changes, sleepless nights, storybooks read, cuddling naps, walk-a-thons, birthday parties, t-ball

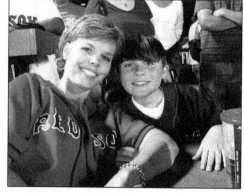

games, writing papers, experiments tested, class fieldtrips, vacations, family time, long chats, proms, relationships, bible studies, praying, singing and rejoicing; our family life has continually evolved from busy days of adventure with great anticipations!

Who knew that the greatest connection in life with you was on the horizon? Who knew that the diagnosis of a devastating muscle disease would bring about our incredible journey of trials, blessings, laughter and tears? Who knew that Duchenne Muscular Dystrophy (DMD) would creep into our world and forge this special bond? Jesus did!

Yes, DMD! Think about it: Where would you and I be *without* this testing of our faith? Only Jesus knows the troubles we've seen, sorrows we've faced, failures we've endured, hardships we've overcome, fears we've encountered, disappointments we've nurtured, wounds we've mended, tears we've cried, questions we've asked, battles we've fought, victories we've won, praises we've extended, new songs we've sung and favor we've received.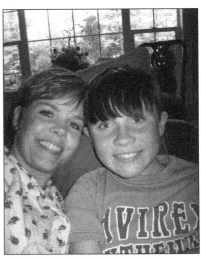

God alone has been our guide, strength, refuge, comfort, joy and peace. The Lord promised to never leave us and He has not. From day one of you being diagnosed, our faithful Savior has held our hands tightly along this unknown path of mystery. All the while He has taught us to love Him deeply, trust Him completely and submit to His call on our lives whether we understand it or not. This disease has had nothing to do with us and everything to do with the Kingdom of Heaven and the Glory of our Lord Jesus Christ.

As I've watched you with family and friends over the years, I've seen you embrace grace, truth, courage, integrity, humor, determination, encouragement, counsel, camaraderie, and energy to persevere your challenges in a profound way. People genuinely love you and have deep respect for your position in life and as a spectator of this disease it blesses my mother's heart to see how you've impacted those around you. Your Dad and I have strived to make your life as normal as possible so others would see *you* and not the disease.

Logan, loving you has made me a much better person. God has guided many of my life's transformations through mothering you. Thank you for the freedoms I have gained by watching the accomplishments you have 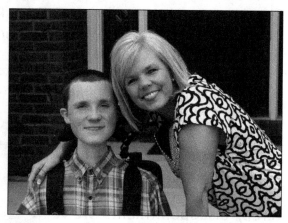 achieved. You are all grown up now and full of God's confidence to be all the Lord wants you to be. Your faithfulness and obedience to our Jesus have inspired me to strengthen my own walk with Him. You are courageous and strong; disciplined and determined; mature and wise; kind hearted and giving; successful and blessed. You are ready for life's next season as this book takes you on new adventures.

Don't you wonder where the Lord may be leading you in all of this? Do you truly realize what you mean to our family? As difficult as this road has been at times, the rewards of becoming stronger, more insightful, understanding and compassionate followers of Christ has been worth it all. The faithfulness of God has brought our family motto to realization; "We may not have it all together, but together (with Jesus) we have it all." We are a winning team!

In closing, you will always hold one of the four designated chambers of my heart. Thank you for all the wonderful memories and may Jesus be the center of all our treasured times yet to come. I will be here for you through this amazing journey. I will love you forever! Like *our* song says: "Winter, spring, summer or fall; all you've got to do is call and I'll be there, yes I will, you've got a friend."

I love you "all the stars in the sky"!
Mommy

Logan's letter to his Dad:

Dear Dad,
 I don't think anything can prepare you to have a son with Duchenne Muscular Dystrophy because, from my understanding, as a dad you expect and want your son to be able to do every-thing that you were able to do. And when I think about it, that must be a lot harder than *being the one* who has DMD because you realized, long before me, what I was missing out on. I can imagine it was and still can be terrible seeing your son unable to experience all the things you love doing! But you haven't let this reality bring forth feelings of bitterness that can only bring harm. I have needed you to grasp that this is the way things are, for now at least, and

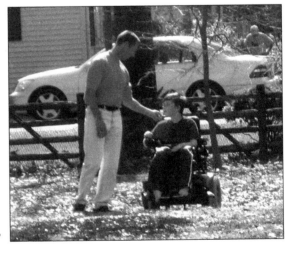

to pass that along to me as a means of encouraging me to do the things I am able to do with excellence. And you have done just that, Dad, even at times where I've been extremely discour-aged. You've encouraged me in a way that has helped me strive to live my life in an impactful manner under the circumstances. You continue to make it clear to me that I can still have a successful and meaningful influence around me, it'll just look a little different than usual.

And in doing this you have always challenged me to do and be the best that I can be, rather than feeling sorry for myself. At the same time, I have needed you to establish and maintain a real hope for the development of a cure for the disease, or even the potential of a miraculous healing because that sort of thing is still possible. It's easier for me to keep this kind of hope, since you do too. In the meantime, as we hope and pray for such a thing to happen, you have always been and even to this day are looking into anything and everything that can and will help with easing the difficulties of Muscular Dystrophy. There is a lot of stuff out there and you're the one that has researched this stuff and worked with me to figure out which things help the best over the years. And I cannot thank you enough for that!

And not to forget mentioning, it has been a huge help (and a miracle in a blessing from God) that your level of expertise and occupation is in physical therapy. This has played a key role in how you have helped me manage everything. We couldn't have made that any better ourselves if we wanted to! I know I couldn't have asked you to do a better job of caring for me in these ways. It took a while longer for me than it probably should have to realize everything that you've always been doing for me. Because it's the only thing I've known, it's just the way things have been all my life. But it means so much to me the more I become aware of it!

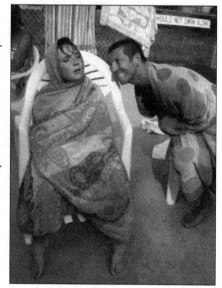

Along with all this, you have always been there to talk with me about all the frustrations I face as I deal with our unique situation. I have needed all the help I can get when it comes to bearing the weight of my daily physical struggles. And you have lead, with little preparation, the entire family in coping with my disability in a phenomenal way. It takes a great leader for a family to become closer through a struggle as great as this, and we've been able to because of an amazing father like you! It definitely adds a whole new dynamic to home life and is a lot harder than what the usual father has to handle, but for some reason you've been chosen to be a DMD dad, and there's no doubt that you have been able to handle it with God's help, and His alone. We are constantly faced with extremely hard, but beneficial, lessons of why and how we must rely on the Lord completely to persevere successfully and you are quick to recognize and help apply them to my life as well as the rest of the family's. We need you! I need you! And I am so thankful for you!

Love, Your Son,
Logan

Now Logan's dad's letter:

My Dear Logan,

You have had quite a journey up to this point in your life. Your journey has also been mine and our family's; and as trials have come and gone, God has been faithful in leading our direction. I rarely wonder how it would be if you were never diagnosed with Duchenne Muscular Dystrophy. When I have pondered that thought, most often it fades quickly because the difficulties that you and our family have had to go through with your condition most always are overshadowed by the blessings. As I work and pray daily on becoming the best possible father, husband, and person I can be, you have been a huge part of my maturity in moving me in the positive direction. We can both be stubborn in our opinions and actions, but we always find a way to move forward.

I remember when you were around 4 years old, and I believe before being diagnosed. We were on vacation and the place we were staying had a pool and behind it a grassy area with sidewalks that went around the grass and led to a deck area and then to the ocean. When exiting the pool, you took the sidewalks to either the right or the left, which rounded the grass area. After a day or two of going from the pool to the ocean and walking the sidewalks, you took off across the grass to get to the deck area. It was basically a straight line to save time and energy. I did not comprehend how much more effort it took you to walk at that time, but you knew it took longer and your mind found a way to compensate. Your physical abilities have been overtaken by this condition, but you have diligently worked your mind to achieve more than most.

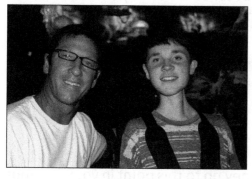

In High School, you set a goal to be Valedictorian and you were determined to follow that through. The homework load was immense especially your Junior and Senior years. You would get home around 2:00 PM – 3:00 PM and work consistently throughout the afternoon and into the night 5, 6, and 7 hours each day.

You would do the same on weekends and most days in the summer due to the Advanced Placement classes. Much of your extra time was due to physical limitations. I can remember you hand writing index cards in such small print, with so much information, and the process taking so much effort and time. Yet you did not want any help. Your condition would allow for certain assistance at school or at home, but you were determined to do everything as any other student would have to do it. Your 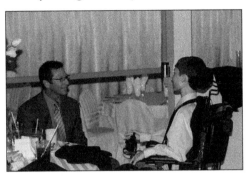 determination was an attribute that was hard not to notice.

What are God's expectations for each of us? I believe many would have different answers and many would have similar answers. But really the only true answer is what God actually expects of us. *"Thou shalt love the Lord thy God with all thy heart, and with all thy soul, and with all thy mind, and with all thy strength."* Mark 12:30. (KJV) Logan you are a 21-year-old young man who has been all boy and now all man. It can be very easy to come to the conclusion that you have missed out on many things because of Duchenne Muscular Dystrophy, and I would agree that is true, but not in the full picture.

Your physical deficits have matured a relationship with God that many people envy. This in itself is worth more than anything that this world can offer. You know Christ as your Savior and you are guaranteed eternal life in heaven. In the Biblical Book of James, it says that life is but a vapor. I know there are some days that don't feel that way, and you and I know there are struggles that you go through that most people really cannot comprehend. I pray for God to heal you and to help us understand His will for your life. I have seen God's fulfillment of his expectations in you and you are an inspiration to me and many others that your life has touched and will touch.

I Love You,
Dad

Logan writes to his older sister:

Dear Sydney,

Because of the gender difference, you and I have not had very many of the same interests, approaches to life, or experiences. But you already knew that! Even though this is true, the relationship between us has been very important. What I've needed from you in the past is just for you to always be willing and ready to come to my aid. Which, for as long as I can remember (though we may clash pretty vehemently and ridiculously sometimes) you have been doing just that. I am so thankful I can count on you for that because I need all the people I can get that are willing to be this sort of help to me! Mom and Dad aren't/won't always be available and because you're the oldest Shannon kid, you've been the next in line to be able to offer help. You have 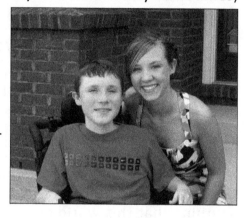 no idea how far your needed selflessness has gone and no idea how much I have appreciated it! I don't always show my gratitude early on or as often as I could/should, but don't let that discourage you because, just like you, I am (and maybe even more so) growing and learning through the process. This is a situation that is testing and trying our entire family, not everyone goes through this and all of us are coming out of it for the better!

You shouldn't be afraid, as I know you aren't, to be an example of working together with patience and love to the important ones around you. Another thing I have needed and RECEIVED from you is for you to reveal what a truly caring and unconditionally loving girl looks like.

Under the circumstances of Muscular Dystrophy, I've gotten to easily see just how shallow and selfish many girls are when it comes to the guys they are attracted to. I know you've seen that just as much as I have. The many girls that I've been interested in have knocked down my interest as if it's nothing; simply because my physical ability and appearance will never meet up to their unreasonable or unattainable expectations. And, like *you know*, that's been rough for me sometimes! At times it has seemed and felt to me like I would never find a girl who will be into me as much as I'm into them. I want them to enjoy me for my personality and not even hold the fact that I have Muscular Dystrophy into consideration. This is part of why you are so important to me and why you are such an amazing big sister. You have definitely

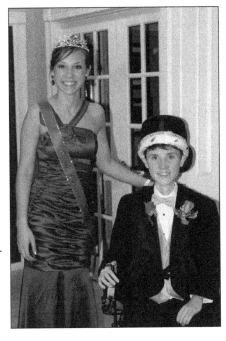

shown the picture to me of what this sort of girl will be like! I can only hope for a girl that resembles you in as many ways as possible! I have always clearly seen that you are completely different than most girls, choosing instead to follow God's pattern of being a woman, meaning you're not all caught up with what's on the surface but rather, what's on the inside. In a very real way, you have continually given me the very real hope that there are other girls out there who are like you and it's only a matter of time before I find one of them. As my sister, you have been a perfect picture of this sort of girl that isn't just beautiful on the outside but on the inside too. So I know that there is another one like you out there. In all reality, to sum up simply and biblically what I've said in this letter I could easily just say you're literally straight out of Proverbs 31 as it spells out how to be this sort of girl, sister etc. I love you so much and I'm so proud to be able to say all of this about my big sis!

Love, Your Brother,
Logan

Logan's sister writes to him:

Logan,

I don't know if I've ever told you 'thank you' in this capacity, but I should have. **Thank you** for being the first human to make me a big sister. **Thank you** for playing on the swing set in the backyard with me. **Thank you** for teaching me about following Jesus. **Thank you** for laughing at my jokes when they aren't lame. **Thank you** for letting me learn how to forgive, after many years of bitterness. **Thank you** for being brave and always sharing what the Lord puts on your heart. **Thank you** for following the Holy Spirit when He prompts you to write/speak. **Thank you** for fighting with me and being quick to apologize. **Thank you** for making my heart sensitive to people who are hurting. **Thank you** for leading your friends in the way of Christ.

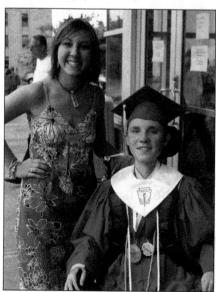

Thank you for making it possible to skip the lines at Disney when we were kids. **Thank you** for having consistent faith that the Lord can and will bring you healing. **Thank you** for being passionate about what you're learning. **Thank you** for persevering through school and work and life. **Thank you** for the days that are fun and the days that are terrible. Mostly, **thank you** for being you.

My life would look drastically different if it weren't for you and Jesus, but if we're being honest – I'm not interested in that life. We have endured many seasons together that have molded us into who we are today and that is the beautiful reality of the faithfulness of our Father. While we don't have answers to all of our questions, we do have the ability to lean on His truth and claim His promises. And that is what you do. As an older sister, I can't help but well up with joy as I watch what you are doing. From sharing the Gospel at graduation to leading Bible studies to writing this book, I am in awe of the ways you are being used. I am so proud of the man you have become and I am honored to call you my brother.

Our family isn't perfect, but it's in our humanness that people see Jesus. Thank you for being such a critical part of that example. You're the best 'oldest of three younger brothers' I could ever ask for.

I love you, for always.
Sydney

Now Logan's letter to his next younger brother:

Dear Devon,
You have always been one of my best friends since as far as I can remember! It has been that way for 20 years of my 21-year life. So as far as friendships go it has been my longest, closest one! With that in mind, I can probably say that 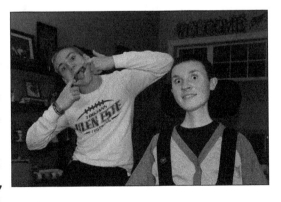 you are my very best friend. That's not to say that I'm not just as much friends with Sydney and Corey, but with the nature of us

both being guys and only being one year apart, it just so happens to be that our sibling relationship is the closest. We have always done everything together, from crazy random antics to playing on sports teams to just about whatever you can name.

We already had years of that in the bag even before I was diagnosed with Duchenne Muscular Dystrophy, which translated to you never considering or realizing that I was ever different. And that has always been the key to how close we are. Perhaps more than any of our peers, you have always known that I am just like everyone else! That's because when we were younger, I was still completely mobile on my own, so at that point there wasn't even a physical difference between the two of us.

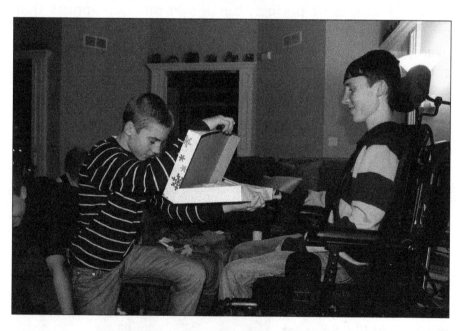

We were able to do the exact same things; and again, were always doing it together. But as we've gotten older, you have always been the one to first notice my getting weaker and slow decline to not be able to do a lot of the things you are able to. I know that had to have been hard for you to watch sometimes, but I've needed *you* to stay strong just as you have needed *me*

to stay strong. I think we've both been able to do that quite well over the years. You have always done your best to be there for me whenever I have needed you to be. We have remained best friends throughout all the highs and deep lows of DMD!

Because my abilities declined over the years, here's a couple of things that went on.... 1) I've spent some time almost looking for some fulfillment of a few dreams *in* you and ***through*** you, especially when it has come to sports. 2) In this, I have cared about you immensely, and believed in you to the point of you being able to do anything that you put your heart to (more than even you believed sometimes). I was that determined to see you successful in the dreams we shared! I know it must have felt like I was being a little too hard on you sometimes with how intense that determination could be; it was just that I know you can do it and so I expect great things out of you!

There's no denying just how much DMD has brought each of us closer together. After me, I've always thought you to be the next person to really understand the change that I've gone through, as we've shared most of our experiences in life ***along-sid***e the other. It differs from a parental relationship.

We may never truly understand why *I* was placed in this circumstance and why ***you*** were simply left to watch me go through it, but both of us are where we are for a reason. So, as you know, we don't need to dwell too much on the why of the ordeal, but instead set our sights on how we can handle and grow from it in the most effective way. I'm glad to say that in the midst of the situation we haven't let the differences that became more and more evident over time outweigh just how much alike we are!

Love You Bro,
Logan

From Devon to his older brother, Logan:

Bro,

It would be impossible for me to include everything inside this letter that you mean to me and how much our relationship has impacted my life. You are my older brother but you are far more than just that to me. You are my hero and my best friend. You mean so much more to me than you will ever know. Through the ups and the downs, and the laughs and the tears, you have been there for me, and I will always be there for you.

We have been sidekicks since day one; whether that meant having fun or getting into trouble. I could not have asked for a better big brother. Logan, your impact on my life is immense. I could never fully express it with words. You have shown me so many things about life and the Christian walk. You have shown me love. You have shown me passion. You have shown me humility. You have shown me faith. You have shown me joy in the midst of pain. You have shown me courage. You have shown me strength. But most of all you have shown me Jesus Christ.

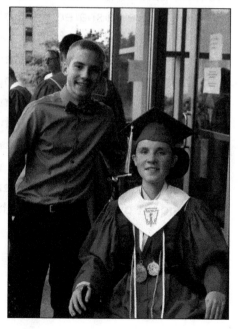

Logan, your life emulates the joy and confidence that we have as Christians and the peace and comfort that Christ brings. The testimony that your life carries is a light in the midst of this ever-darkening world. Although we both know that you are far from perfect and that your situation has been far from a breeze, you still, through it all, never stopped being the Godly example that I look up to. You hunger and you thirst after God's Word and His promises.

This example drives me to grow closer to God every day. I hope to someday have as much passion for our Savior that you have in your pinky finger. I do not comprehend how anyone could look at your life and not see the truth that Christ changes lives. I look around and I see all those out there who have personal vendettas toward God because misfortune has fallen on their life or the world is suffering, but they don't realize that **you have just as much of a right** to think like that; yet you don't. You don't curse God for having DMD; instead you do your best to praise Him through it. I know that everyone who reads this book will get something different out of it, but I also know that each and every person will see the light of Christ that is in you. From the time we were kids I always wondered why God chose you to have DMD instead of me, or why you even had it at all, but now I see that He knew you would be strong enough to fight and that you would make an everlasting impact for Him in the lives of all those around you. I praise God for you and I thank Him for allowing me to share this life journey with you, Log.

I have so much more I could say to you but I think that would take a book in itself, so I will close with this. I love you Logan. I will always love you and I will always be here for you. Do not ever stop showing the love of Christ to all those you encounter. You are the strongest and most courageous person that I will ever know. I am so proud to call you my big brother.

Love,
Devon

Logan writes some thoughts about his youngest brother, Corey:

Dear Corey,
To have a big brother with Duchenne Muscular Dystrophy is to be in a very unique position. Because muscular dystrophy is a

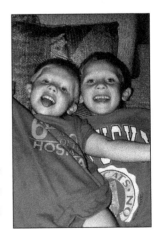

degenerative disease, and it slowly gets a little worse over time until we eventually usually become wheelchair ridden, that has meant you've had an older brother that has virtually always been less physically able than you. That is by no means an average or normal situation. And yet, because of the nature of our family, you have always realized that I am just like everyone else, which we can be thankful for!

With our scenario being considerably different from the one between Devon and I; much, really all, of the time we spent together has involved a major ability difference. So, even though we've spent just as much time with each other as our other siblings, whenever we have been or are together, it has required a lot of your helping me. In many ways, that is entirely opposite of the typical big brother/little brother relationship. And you know what, that's kind of weird, but we've probably done just as well with it as any pair of brothers could! I am so thankful for the way that we've always been able to handle such an odd circumstance! We have always been there for each other in the way that we are able and/or needed to be, even if it takes a little longer to get to that point sometimes. And I really hope that you can agree. Just as I have been guilty of doing this with Devon, I've looked for some fulfillment of lost dreams in you and through you.

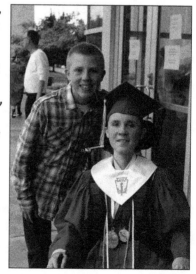

Sometimes it has been with sports, but more so with you it has been with music and singing ability as we are basically equally talented, but the fact is you just happen to have far better lung "functionability." Rather than being bitter about it, I'm good with relinquishing it and cheering you on to excellence in that category instead.

So it goes without saying that I care exceedingly about you and know that you are capable of some truly great things! I hope that you have never felt like I'm being too hard on you or have way too high expectations, because I can see how that might be. It is just that I know you can do it and can't help but expect amazing things from you! And while we're on the topic, one of my favorite parts of our relationship has and always will be when we are singing together! There's no denying just how close the difficulties of DMD have brought us together as brothers. And there will always be questions as to why our lives have gone this way, but we don't need to dwell too much on those "whys", but instead set our sights on how we can handle it to the glory of God!

Love, Your Big Brother,
Logan

Corey writes to his oldest brother, Logan:

Dear Logan,
Eighteen years have passed in my life and you've been there through all of them (obviously). Although those years have been painful, and sometimes a struggle, there's no way I would want God to change what He's blessed me with – a brother whose heart and mind for the Lord is too big to be contained by the four walls of our house. So, I'm glad you had to write a book to share some of that knowledge, grace, and wisdom with the world.

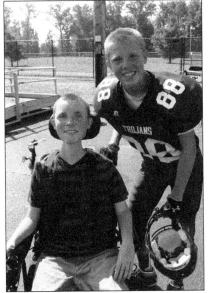

To point out a specific memory that stands out isn't something easy to do for me. Even though I was alive while you could walk, those days have escaped my mind, except for a few snippets of scenes: riding bikes, throwing action figures in trees and you tripping and falling down Christmas morning before we reached the living room. I feel like no matter what I say in this letter, I will never completely be able to explain to others the bond that our family, and specifically, that you and I share. The number of tears I've cried in the past wanting you so badly to walk and run with me, are innumerable. I didn't know why God wouldn't give you muscles that would support you, and I was so confused. I didn't know what to think except to just try to go with the flow. It wasn't easy trying to understand why our family was put into this situation and why we had to be given all this to carry on our shoulders.

All of these thoughts were amplified at the time of your scoliosis surgery and the amount of time I had that summer to think about everything. I was scared, but I didn't really show it because I felt like I had to stay strong for you so that you wouldn't be scared. During that summer, I had to trust God like never before. I felt deep inside that I had to trust Him to keep you alive. With my level of understanding as a sixth grader, I searched and wasn't for sure that the outcome would be positive. I've tried to completely understand it all; why we're still in this situation, and feel I know I never will. And I'm okay with that. Our path as a family, with Duchenne Muscular Dystrophy at its center, has brought me to the point of surrender to God that I experience today. I've put your healing, our family, and my life in God's hands, and I doubt I'd be at this same point in my walk with Jesus if it wasn't for the situation we're in.

I know it isn't easy at all to live without the physical ability to do things, and how annoying it is for you to go through the painstaking process it is to make yourself comfortable in your chair every day. Although my patience dies quickly at times, I want you to know that I love you, and I want to thank you for what you are to me. A brother who, although can't walk, sprints towards God's will for his life full speed ahead! I thank God for the family I've been given, and a brother that loves me enough to mention me in his book ;).

But for real, God's using us both, and it's amazing to see His hand moving us to great places to serve Him.

Never forget that He has got it all under control. I mean He is THE ONE and ONLY GOD. He's a pretty big deal. I love you, Logan.

Love,
Corey

And this wraps up Logan's letters with his family. You can see how letters can do wonders to lift the spirits of those who have faced hardships and tragedies. When Logan and I were talking, we discussed how these letters could actually be like a model for someone else to send a grateful acknowledgement of someone's care, service, and love. It could be a family member or a close friend, a cousin, or even a co-worker. But recognizing people that have reached out to us when we have experienced pain and loss is so important, yet frequently overlooked. Floods carry away homes, tornadoes level entire communities, a plane crash can claim a precious life so early, and a misunderstanding in a family can fester as a cancer until it's settled. So why not write someone today? A text has its place. A phone call has its place. But a letter or a personal visit retains a value that is among diamonds and rubies. The Lord smiles when we reach out to others. Try it now…….

Chapter 15 – Intermission #2

What's "Seen", What's "Behind the Scenes" and What's "Needed"

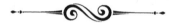

As we take another break from the collection of letters, comments and deep thoughts, what if we took a few moments to unveil some special, tender, and revealing insight into this special Shannon family? Michael and Tyra are the parents, and Sydney is the eldest child and only daughter. Logan is second and the oldest son. Devon is third and Corey is the youngest. They live in a nice single-level home that was built for that sized family, with special considerations included because of Logan's mobility situation. The lot they chose is adjacent to the Glen Este middle school and high school campuses, with the rear portion of their property actually bordering the school

"The generosity and affection of some residents in their neighborhood allowed a concrete driveway to be built for Logan so he could drive his wheelchair himself to school on decent days without having to be driven to school and back home again each day."

property. (The current facility is in the process of combining with another school and relocated to a newer, larger campus.)

The generosity and affection of some residents in their neighborhood allowed a concrete walkway to be built for Logan so he could drive his wheelchair himself to school on decent days without having to be driven to school and back home again each day. The walkway was built from one corner edge of the school parking lot to the top end of two driveways near the houses next door. He would take off from his house, go down his driveway into the cul-de-sac, go up the neighbor's driveway all the way up to the end where the special concrete walkway started, and take that walkway to the school parking lot.

In the summer, Logan would try to dodge mosquitoes and other predatory insects with his illusive and resourceful acrobatic maneuvers, to the disgust of those insects that were denied a meal. On autumn days, the falling leaves would dance around him as he and his brother(s) and sister would head to the school. In spring, the fragrance of blooming bulbs, fresh green leaves, and fruit trees would waft through the air, spilling a divine aromatic nectar into the wind during the brief travel to school. In winter, different dedicated snow shovelers would make the path open for Logan as the wheelchair sought to maintain traction. That would make anyone watching smile.

> *"In winter, different dedicated snow shovelers would make the path open for Logan as the wheelchair sought to maintain traction. That would make anyone watching smile."*

On those rainy days, umbrellas would pop out. Of course, in really bad weather, there was always the option of being transported in the Shannon's specially equipped mini-van with ramp and securing device. But there were always friends around at school that would render assistance for Logan when he needed it. This was a testimony to his character, and how his behavior and faith structure actually built a personal and loyal group of people around him. And people **wanted** to be part. If some students were in class with Logan, they would make sure he got to the class OK. Like a lion pride takes care of its own.

The Shannons are so similar to all of us, because they have bills to pay, groceries to buy, sports events to go to, errands to run, vacations to take, squabbles to disperse, sicknesses to treat, chores to do, repairs and maintenance to be done on cars and home, scrapes and cuts to put bandages on, birthday and graduation parties to go to, etc. I could go on and on.

We may have different vacation destinations; we may have different bills to pay; we may like different sports teams; we may have different jobs or go to different churches; but we can easily identify with things this family has to do as a normal routine.

Do we sometimes feel that we have struggles that others may not be having? Do we sometimes believe that no one would possibly understand what we're going through?

> *"The Shannons are so similar to all of us, because they have bills to pay, groceries to buy, sports events to go to, errands to run, vacations to take, squabbles to disperse..."*

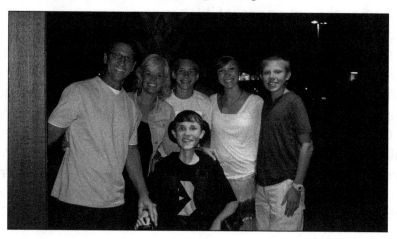

Someone once said that if a group of us could put our problems into a central pile with all the contributors circling the large pile, we would be so surprised at what heavy loads others are carrying; that we'd pick our own back up without a single complaint or grumble.

What if **this second intermission** was broken into three categories? We all know from our own lives that there are things we see, things that aren't seen by others, and things we'd like to see and be seen.

A) **What is "seen" by observation**

B) **What is "behind the scenes" meaning not normally seen**

C) **What we "need" because we now understand**

So what is "seen"? It is simply what we can perceive and measure through our senses. What can we learn about ourselves as we look at the Shannons going forward?

I want you to think about something. When we see different people out in public, do we think about what kind of a life that person is really living? Do we allow our imaginations to fill in the "blanks" about people before we know anything about them? Do we allow our past experiences to cloud or screen our current opinions? Do we assume that by watching a few fleeting moments, we can conclude a total situation or condition?

"When we see different people out in public, do we think about what kind of a life that person is really living?"

For instance, when we see a young pre-teen boy in a wheelchair trying to reach some audio equipment in a store, what do we think?

Do we automatically assume he was born that way?

Do we automatically assume the family was hit broadside by a drunk driver?

Do we automatically assume he was adopted because no one wanted him?

The real issue is that the young pre-teen boy is a person; who is living inside a body that requires a wheelchair. And we need to view that person **past** what we "see".

When we see an older lady pulling a portable oxygen bottle on a cart with an air line running to her face trying to shop at a grocery store, what do we really "see"?

Do we automatically assume she was a chain smoker, and she is now having to deal with the choices she made?

Do we automatically assume she was in a factory job where she was exposed to high levels of dangerous air-born materials?

The real issue is that the older lady is a person; who is living in a body that has a need for oxygen. We need to view that person **past** what we "see".

Seen at Home (with the Shannons)

Logan zips around the house in his wheelchair, and can go outside if someone opens the door. He is eager to be going through his quiet time and devotionals by himself or be part of other conversations.

He converses with ease, even in larger crowds visiting his home; and his smile is contagious.

He joins in the chatter of his family and friends when groups show up.

He can get into serious discussions about sports, faith, government, family, relationships, finance issues, and education when those topics become the conversation.

He breaks into song when he hears ones he likes. And he has a good voice. With his lung capacity affected by DMD, the volume isn't there. But the passion and pitch is right on!

When eating, someone has to be there to feed him.

Logan takes prayer time seriously, and knows God has a special path ahead. He doesn't know why he's been assigned this road through life, but he knows something's up. He is a man. He is smart. He is capable.

He is part of the family. He teases and he gets teased. He jokes and gets joked on. As a family, the Shannons like to watch their favorite sports teams, and cheer for their favorite players!

Sometimes, there would be crowds of folks with the same team loyalties, and that inside crowd reaction to calls or scoring would be just like if you were there! With them being part of the Glen Este school system (which is part of the West Clermont [Ohio] school system), the Shannons frequently attend local games where they have a family member on one of the teams. Sydney excelled at women's volleyball, Devon and Corey were on the men's football teams, and Logan was there being a big part in the cheering section, zipping up and down the sidelines in his wheelchair "chariot". The crowd was always involved and accepted *all* the Shannons as part of their fan fabric.

Seen Out and About

Someone near Logan's home might see him enjoying different musical events and concerts when taken by family or friends. He likes music that lifts up people's hearts and soothes deep hurts and pains, and brings real life situations into focus.

He goes to sports events and professional sports stadiums or arenas, and takes in all the action. He rides with family or friends when he goes, and enjoys the banter going to the event and coming home from the event. Logan favors wearing clothes from his favorite pro teams.

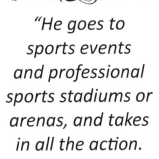

"He goes to sports events and professional sports stadiums or arenas, and takes in all the action. He rides with family or friends when he goes, and enjoys the banter going to the event and coming home from the event."

He goes to restaurants sometimes with family or friends, and they cut up the food or lift the drink for Logan.

When transported in the specially equipped van, Logan can go shopping at malls, at individual stores or even grocery stores if he wants. We went to graphic designers, had meetings with printers, and had pictures made at an establishment by one of the photographers.

If he sneezes, who holds the handkerchief? Who holds it while he blows the rest out of his nose? Someone has to. Gross? Maybe to some... But a friend will be there. Family will be there. Because they see the person.

When he has to use the restroom, how does he take care of that? Who helps?

When he wants to shop for new threads, who needs to help get something off the rack?

When he wants to work on his iphone, who lifts his hands up from the wheelchair arm rests to the table where the iphone is located?

When he was in high school at cafeteria time – who fed Logan? Who cut his food?

Who opened his locker? How did he carry his books?

How did he get a drink of water? He couldn't push any button on the water fountain.

If he wants to answer a question, how does he get the teacher's attention since he can't raise his hand?

How does he take tests? How does he hold a pen or pencil?

When we strictly go by what we "see" by Logan himself it is so different than "seeing" Logan with so many friends and family who give of themselves for a healthy person who happens to be in a wheelchair.

What's Behind the Scenes

So what does "behind the scenes" mean anyway?

It doesn't have to be intentional, but some things are better left private, others are simply nobody's business, and others are special occasions meant to remain between the parties involved.

1) What does it take to make sure Logan looks great and presentable? We **all** want to look good when we get ready to go somewhere. We choose what's appropriate for a particular occasion, and we wear that. Since Logan can't get ready himself, all that preparation has to be done by someone else or with someone else. Logan may recommend an outfit, but others have to put it on. We don't make things public as we get ready. It's not seen.

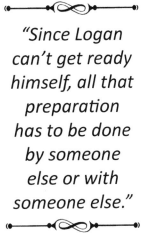

"Since Logan can't get ready himself, all that preparation has to be done by someone else or with someone else."

2) When we have to eat, and eat on a regular basis; we just do it, right? But when Logan eats, someone else has to prepare it, someone else has to take it out of the pots and pans and put it on a plate, someone has to cut it up into smaller sizable chunks, someone else has to season it to his own individual taste, and then someone else has to feed Logan. And "feeding" means to use utensils to move the food to his open mouth. It means the right amount, because chewing requires muscles, and the rate of chewing and swallowing **_has_** to be considered. It just can't be shoveled in like some of these crazy food shows. Logan can't consume food like Adam Richman on Travel Channel's "Man vs. Food" show used to! And we all know that when we eat, we have to have something refreshing to wash it all down. We've all been there right?! But we know when to take a drink, and we know how fast to gulp. But Logan has to ask someone to hold up a beverage so

he can use the straw to enjoy it. And he also has to stop drinking to tell you he's had enough; and someone has to be aware of that in order to pause and let Logan say if he wants another sip or not. Unless that's at a restaurant somewhere, it's not seen.

3) When it's time to use the restroom, we excuse ourselves, get up, take care of business, and return. What does Logan do? What **can** Logan do? He has to ask for someone to help him in that area, too. Gravity helps every person in digestion. It is no different with Logan. But in his case, gravity is basically the only thing. Although we have muscles for control, Logan is losing his. He informs the responsible member that he needs to use the bathroom, and someone else has to help him. It's behind the scenes. After he's done, Logan returns into public view.

4) When we prepare to get up out of bed, or when we prepare to go to bed, we just do it. But Logan needs 100% assistance. Is that bad? No. It's just reality. Logan cannot get out of bed, cannot shave or brush his teeth or comb his hair, and cannot dry himself after a shower and put his clothes on. Someone has to help him. Without helping, Logan doesn't get up, get ready, get dressed, or get fed. It's behind the scenes.

5) When Logan wants to read, someone has to get the book, open the book, and turn the pages. We don't even think about all those steps. We just do it. When was the last time you liked something you read and went back because a particular thing caught your attention a few chapters ago? You simply turned back. Logan has to ask to turn back to see a particular section again. It's unseen. Now, Logan does operate a mobile device (smart phone) with some success. But still, someone has to physically move his arms from the arms of the wheelchair, and place them up on a countertop or a table where he can use his limited hand and finger functions to participate in the

outside world. But if he wants to move the wheelchair around, he needs someone to move his arms back onto the arms of the wheelchair and position his right hand ever so carefully around the joystick control. Then Logan is ready. But usually not seen.

Once I touched Logan's right hand at a local football game as a greeting. With the slightest touch, it moved the joystick unintentionally and I **_ran over my own foot_** with the immense weight of that wheelchair! The joystick controller was so sensitive! Logan was as surprised as I was, but then had a grin on his face that told me, "You knew better than to do that!" (And I did know better, I just got careless!)

6) When Logan shows up at church, at the mall, at a concert, at a play or out on the town with friends or family, someone has to drive him there. He doesn't just show up. He waits. When everyone else is ready, then he goes. Sometimes we just take all of the steps to go somewhere without even thinking of it! Logan **thinks** of those steps, and can't just **do** them. He **has** to wait on whoever will be responsible for the transportation. People usually just see Logan there.

God takes care of us as a caring Father, just like when parents take care of infants or those who have no other way of surviving. God watches over us like parents watch over their children, no matter what age. Note the parallel of God taking care of us with **His** abilities and Logan's parents taking care of him with **their** abilities. We "needed" our parents with their protection, with their maintenance, and their provisions when we were young. With all that said, it's evident a whole lot of work goes into what everyone sees when Logan shows up looking dapper!

So I want to bring some people from behind the scenes, and whisk the spotlight on them for a moment during this intermission. Logan's family deserves some time.

Sydney – is a brilliant older sister who is a fierce defender of Logan. She has grace and poise, and is a real lady. She has a deep faith in God, and she has a heart for helping people. Whether it is on a mission trip to Australia or lending a hand to strangers, Sydney knows that the right attitude has everything to do with how she lives.

In high school, she was on the school volleyball team, and was a force to be dealt with on the court. Yet, she had kindness with those she dealt with. She watched over Logan when she could and helped with Logan when she could at school and with their mom after they got home.

Sydney graduated a valedictorian from high school, and then as summa cum laude from Lipscomb University.

She got married in 2016, and her husband, Wynton, is the brother of Logan's best friend, Macon.

Devon – is on the quiet side, except his sense of humor bursts forth with his family. He is about a year younger than Logan, and steps in to help, as well. Logan and Devon are close and wrestled around back in the early days. There would be those times when rough housing would be the preferred passing of time. Since the Shannon family likes sports, there are always discussions about team strength, standings in the different divisions, and favorite teams like the Red Sox, the Patriots, the Celtics and the Bruins.

Devon is also very smart, and graduated a valedictorian from high school, as well. He played football in high school, and is not a stranger to dedicating himself to tasks. So helping with Logan is natural for him. This brotherly love and support is vital to helping share the load. Devon's faith in God is also demonstrated in character, in speech, and in life; and that is following him as he goes into the medical field.

Corey – is the youngest brother and sibling, and is three years younger than Devon.

Corey helps with outside work, and occasionally takes care of Logan while Mom is running errands, etc. He also was on the football team, but changed to track this last year. He also plays actively on the tennis team. Intelligence didn't stop with Devon, because Corey is also on track to graduate a valedictorian. And like the rest of the family, he has been growing in his faith, as well.

Corey also excels in business applications and was 5th in the nation when competing in a business role play when presented with assumptions and directives to find a profitable solution!

Michael – is Logan's Dad, and has an important management position in a sports rehabilitation and physical therapy company, and has skills from that field to provide Logan vital home relief from Duchenne Muscular Dystrophy issues. But Michael yearns to provide for his family, although work-related tasks pressure him into longer hours. The complexity of health-care regulations has saddled providers across the board with an increase in a seemingly unending load of paperwork and documentation, which also adds pressure to everyone. But don't let his quiet demeanor be seen as weakness. He's tough, but accessible, because he has some flexibility to work from home on occasion.

There is always a precarious balancing act that takes place where there just aren't enough hours in the day to divide between the high-pressure management stuff, the things at home that need tending to, the personal things at home with his family that will continue to strengthen the bonds, the special things with Logan that Michael **wants** to do, and to spend time with each loved one at home. Other things also need to be crowded into the jammed schedule like recreational activities, sports activities, vacations, special events like birthdays, graduations, funerals, anniversaries, reunions, emergencies, special acts of kindness, and you have a recipe for stress that could break a man.

But Michael has his faith in Christ. He has a dependence on the truth of the Scriptures. He knows that Jesus Christ is faithful in working in the lives of believers as we go along the rock-strewn paths; guiding us through storms of life, keeping our heads clear, and vision focused forward. He accepts the inner strength that the Lord allows him to have to see and meet the needs of his family.

Initial suspicions that Michael saw in Logan's early troubles didn't prepare him for what was to follow. How do you react to a looming medical possibility? Was it temporary, or not? Many things cross our minds. Could it be dealt with by special prescriptions? Would Logan grow out of this? Michael kept thinking about his growing family in a new light. What if his other sons would have similar physical challenges? It had to have crossed his mind that with this disease, he'd never be able to play catch with Logan. But he would make up for it. He prayed for answers.

Back when Logan was young, Michael and his wife, Tyra, found out what was happening to their oldest son. They could never imagine how expensive all the necessary support equipment was going to be. It began to mount up, even though insurance coverage provided partial relief. As time went on, Michael had to begin factoring in how the family budget could sustain an ever-increasing drain on finances. The kids were growing, which meant larger food bills and money being set aside for college. There were also elderly grandparents who would be relying more on their children for higher levels of assistance. Here again, Michael's faith would supply the answer. God not only IS everything, He OWNS everything. During those deeply emotional prayer times, Michael would trust his God, and fully understand that He does supply **_all_** our needs. And God has not been slack in His provisions. Michael has seen incredible examples of things working out.

So what would **_you_** do in this situation? What should **_he_** do in this situation? While it is tough to place ourselves in other people's lives, it's easier to place them on our personal prayer lists, as I have Michael. We all recognize stress in others, and we are obligated to take part of that load as fellow believers.

Michael has shown his faith by being part of fund-raisers, positioning himself and his family to major motivational speakers like Zig Ziglar to draw attention to needs of many people with challenges and disabilities. This awareness brings people together in a wonderful way, and the Lord is using him as the person who understands this key motivational part.

Because Michael comes into contact with many, many people during the course of a day, he has access to opinions, recommendations, great counsel, and experience from countless others. His days are filled with meetings, new interviews and hires, resolution of conflict, training on new software, explanations of new processes, studying new equipment and procedures, and teleconferencing with branch offices and home offices.

Would anyone think that this position would be the one he dreamed about when he was young? In those times between the hectic schedules, does he wonder about what else he could be doing? He reflects on how much more he could be doing for Logan to give Tyra a break. Does he regret any part of his life because all this complication has been placed in his path? Because of the unseen aspects of anyone's life, we can all be sure that no one's life is absolutely what they expected.

Michael is no different. Would he like to play tackle football with Logan? Would he like to rough house with all of his boys? Sure! So Michael adjusts the ways that he can. In private moments, he thinks about the Lord, and how all this came to be. He prays about how to pray. He prays about his whole family. He prays about his son, Logan, and what the future will hold. He smiles because Logan has become a man. He knows the Lord has answered his prayers. He looks to the future, because God is already there.

Tyra – is Logan's Mom, and a genuine possessor of a servant's heart. As a young mom, she envisioned her growing family in her mind and heart. We've all had those dreams and plans, haven't we? Really, how often do we see troubles and storms ahead?

Sometimes, but not always. There always seems to be sudden changes in our lives, and we need to roll with them. How many times have we taken steps to shove the difficulties and hazards away from our families, especially our children? What we **don't** expect is being blind-sided by a calamity that appears to sneak up on us by surprise. With Tyra being home and watching her children, she began to notice things about Logan's growing physical difficulties. Questions went through her mind. As time went on, she and Michael discussed the situation and options. And at no time, did things proceed without prayer. They lifted their children up in prayer and asked the Lord for His guidance and direction.

You can ask them if God supplied the answers they were looking for. Did God promise them He'd "fix" things up? Did God jump in and make everything OK? As the family prayed, some would think the Lord dismissed those prayers, because Logan's condition became worse. But Michael and Tyra trusted in God's will. Do we look at what's *seen* by a physical condition more than what's *unseen* as a development of a character, a molding of a life, and a fulfillment of a destiny? Do we see Logan's declining physical condition as the answer God wanted? Was this supposed to happen this way? How does a person check whether this is true or not? How do we know? Are we **supposed** to know?

Tyra would seek the Lord and the counsel of trusted friends about what was happening. Her heart would yearn for a solution that would allow a complete recovery. But her strong faith would take her to a level of understanding that would position her as a powerful source of strength for others! As she grew in her faith in Jesus Christ, that passion would fuel growth in others as her children grew. It would end up being an unknown gift to many others, where they would seek her for **their** hour of need, to gain strength. It would be a time that she didn't see coming, but she'd be there as a living example that others could see of how to cope, how to endure, how to hold on.....

Would this be easy? No. As time went on, she had to do more and more for Logan. He became weaker and weaker. Sydney, Devon, and Corey were brought gradually into the knowledge of their brother's condition, with the instruction that they'd be required to help out in an increasing way down the road. Any assistance would be assigned according to what the need was, but reminders were constant that Logan was THEIR brother, and if roles were different, he would be in on the team that would do the same thing for them.

Logan's room was equipped with an audible monitoring device that would relay any noises from Logan's room to the master bedroom. When Logan would stir at night, Tyra was the one who typically would get up and respond to what the issue was. Her ears became tuned to the slightest sounds. It was like she was constantly on high alert with her internal radar always sweeping the acoustic horizon, listening for those sometimes imperceptible stirrings of a loved one. Can't get much rest that way, so it can take its toll.

There are other consequences and sacrifices that are unseen. Tyra loves people. I have seen her at her children's parties at home and other places where people will gather. I have seen so many pictures of graduation activities and the energy all those young people bring wherever they congregate! She loves to mingle, and has the ability to either navigate purely cavalier conversations or have deep, meaningful, powerful and life-changing exchanges. She has a sensitivity about others that is truly a spiritual gift. There is a man who is up in years who goes to our church and he has a debilitating arthritic condition. She made many visits to his home before his wife passed away because she has that kind of heart. Now the man's wife has passed away, and Tyra keeps visiting. She **ministers** to people.

As Tyra touches lives, she is also affected; she sees changes where she's left her prints. Jesus Christ has groomed her and molded her into a servant of His love. The Lord uses the ripples from her pond to affect things far away in a positive way. When she weeps, there is a tendency to keep that private. But when it's time to rejoice, let's make sure that's public!

But what about her, personally? Did she or does she have dreams of her own? Were her early creative reaches cut short because of all the necessary and time-consuming attention needed for Logan? What were the things she thought about doing long ago that she was never able to do? Did she willingly sacrifice for her family's needs while slowly releasing her grip on that dream? There is something inside Tyra that has a strong undercurrent. Like Michael, she has an embrace of God's power and principles from the Scriptures that allows her to sink deep roots into His understanding. They might apply it differently, but they seek God's blessing with their hearts.

But Tyra **has** actually lived her dream. *I would like to paraphrase the final scene of Mr. Holland's Opus,* a movie starring Richard Dreyfuss, with Tyra's influence. "...look around. There isn't a life here that hasn't been touched. Each person is a better one because of you. We are your 'symphony'. We are the melodies and notes of your presence, and we are the music of your life."

Imagine all the energy of school kids stopping in after school to see Logan and his siblings, the wonderful chaos of kids having a fun time! The laughs, the practical jokes, the food fights, the nights when the rooms were packed watching the big game, the chugging down the food and rushing out the door when things were running late. Imagine Tyra's threatening finger pointing at someone who dared to violate one of the "rules", wearing a scowl that would put fear into the hearts of organized crime members. And then as she rounded a corner into another room, she would break out into a smile that would light up Cincinnati.

She was molding all these young lives step by step, moment by moment; all the time caring for Logan and the rest of her children. It was an intentional **investment** into her children's lives and an ancillary investment into all the lives around her. Her faith and the extended influence of it is not sequestered to folks only located in the Southwest Ohio, Northern Kentucky region, either.

Lately, Sydney has completed college and Devon is in college. The endless parade of youth has diminished substantially, and things are much quieter now. Although more time must be spent caring for Logan, and the level of youthful activities has waned, there are still things that need to be done. What happens in those hours? When the kids were showing up, the parents would more often show up. But as the numbers of children fall, one side effect is that less people come to visit.

Tyra has a life to give, and she has shown character, resilience and resoluteness in doing that. And she's not done yet!

What's Needed

People have a desire to be needed. We need to feel we have value, even though God has expressly stated that He made each one of us for a particular purpose in this world. Yes, we need food, but feeling wanted and needed has been determined to be a deep emotional requirement.

So **when** can we give back? **How** do we give back? Sometimes a card or letter really helps those who are doing the same things over and over with life-giving assistance to one in need. Prayers provide amazing results as we lift up those concerns to a holy God, and allow Him to administer blessings. Write out prayers and send them!

When we text, IM, face time, etc., etc.; it's gone pretty quickly. But when we take the time to actually write out a heart-felt message of love, of encouragement, or of inspiration; it can be re-read over and over, bringing new hope each time.

If you want to really be an uplifting presence to one who is constantly caring for a close family member or friend, spend time with them! Invest in helping them make their other com-mitments and obligations. **Anyone** can do this. YOU can do this. Do errands or make a quick meal or bring in some lunch, assist in someone's kids' homework or sports practices, or just be there for some cool conversation! But love them!

Logan's family and friends have already shown how they do it; and they're not done yet!!

So grab another cup of coffee or tea and settle in....

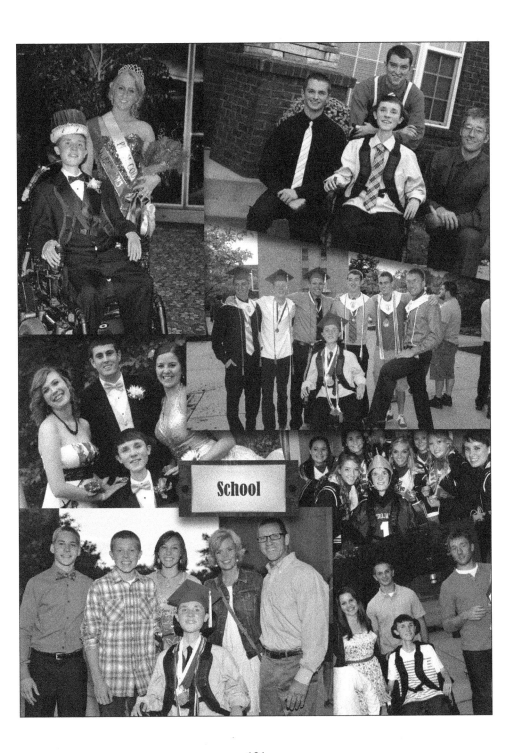

School

181

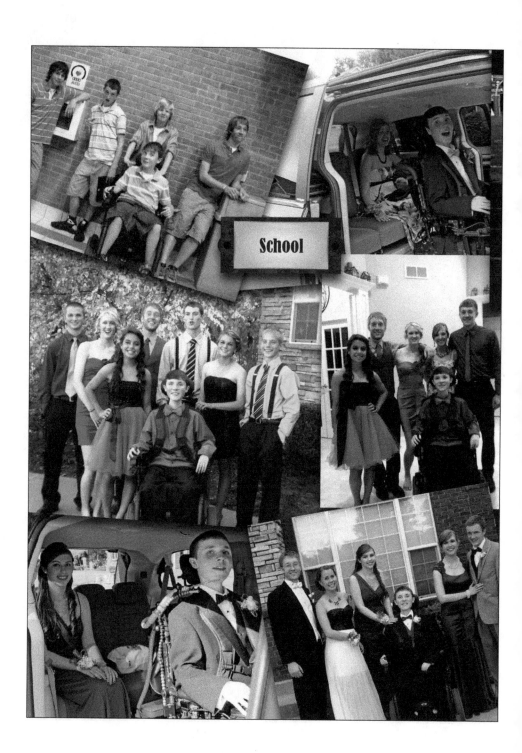

School

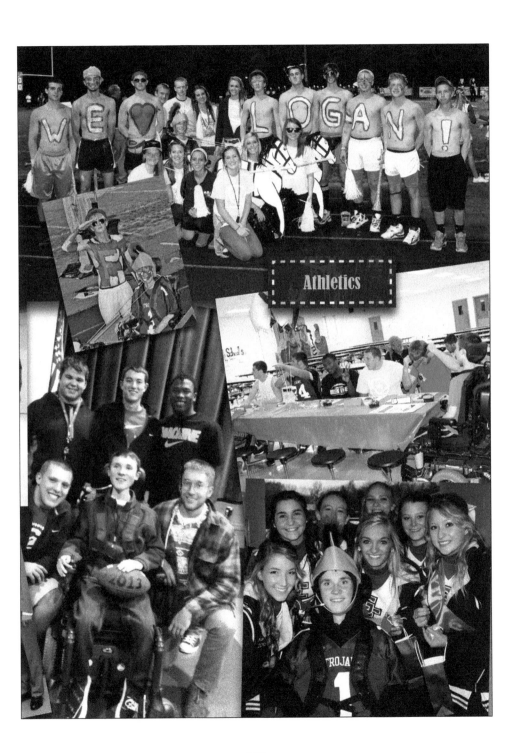

Athletics

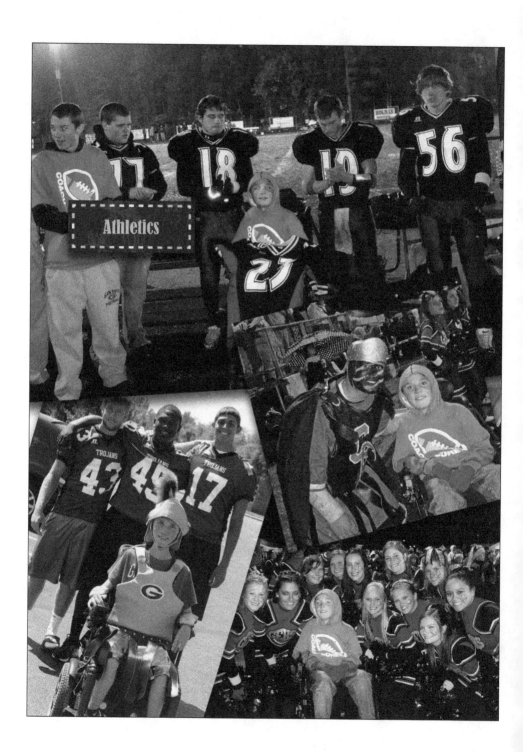

Athletics

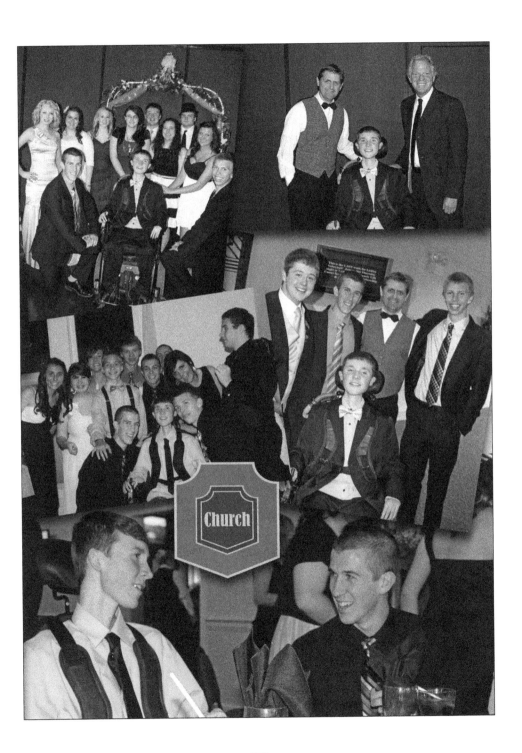

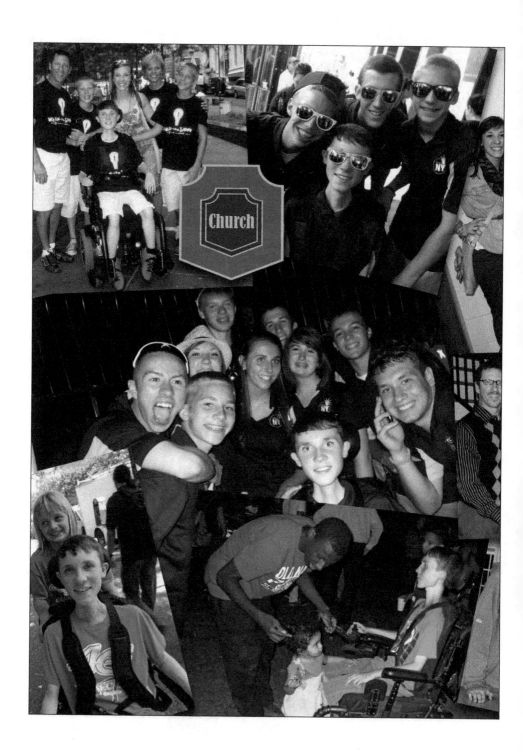

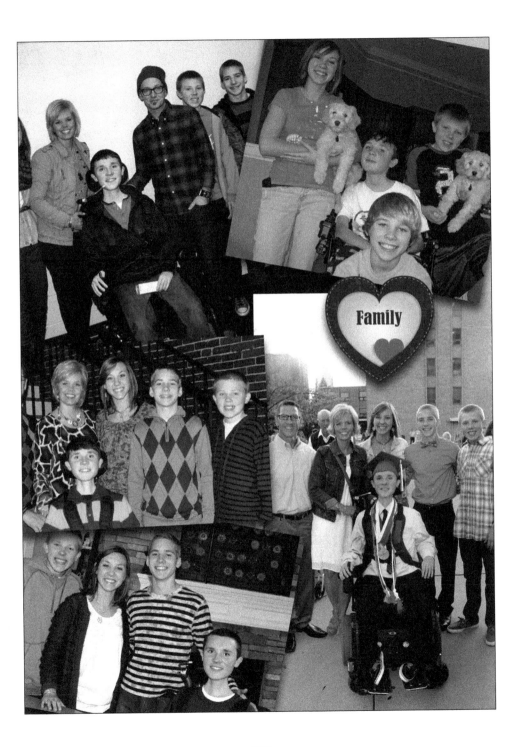

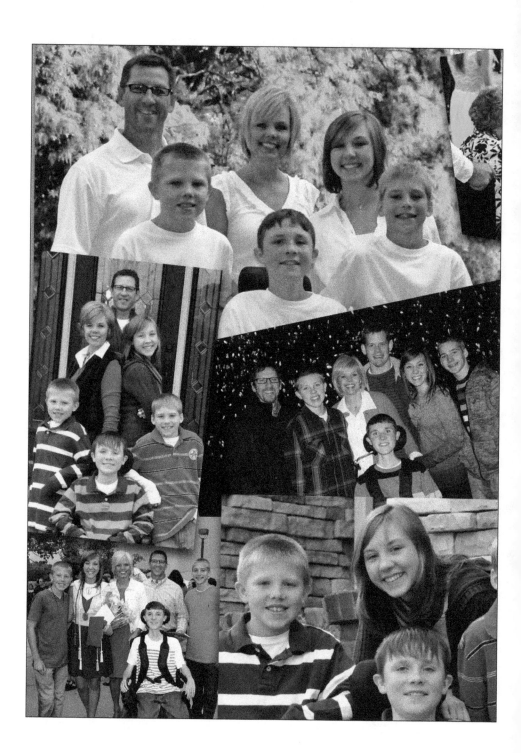

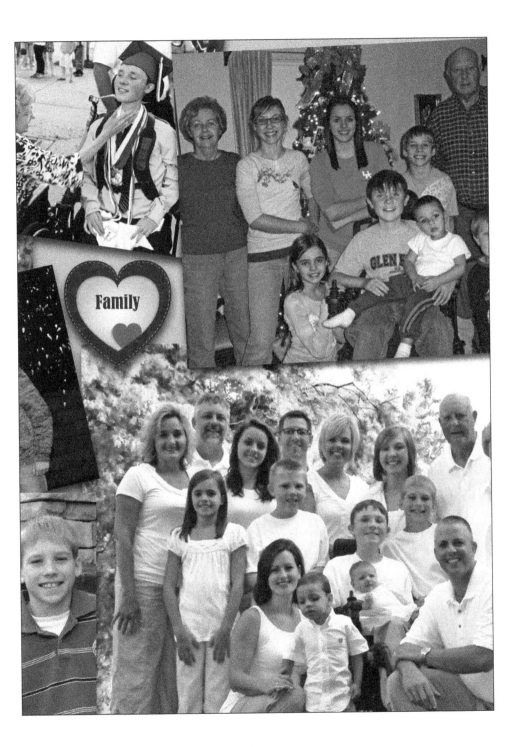

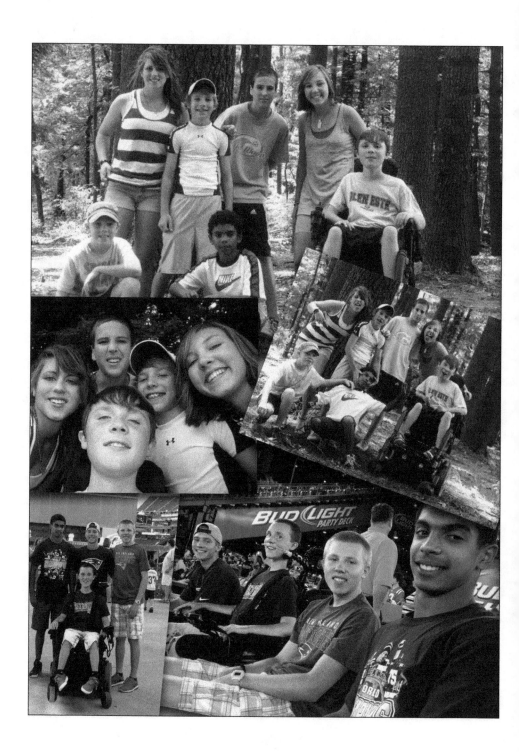

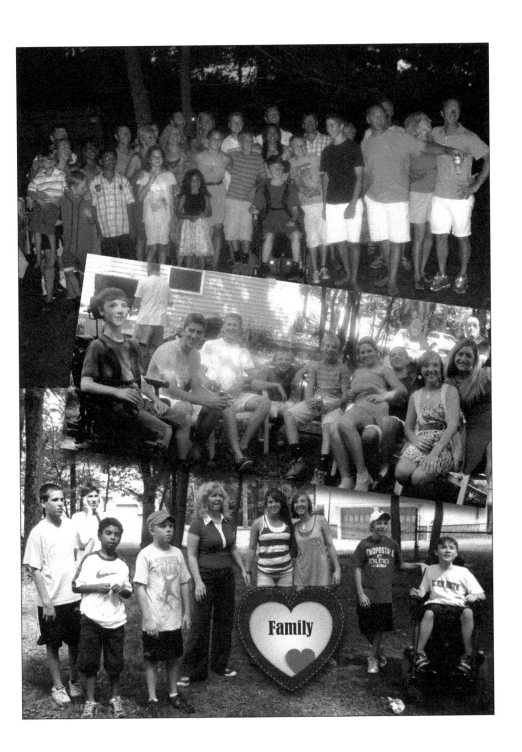

Family

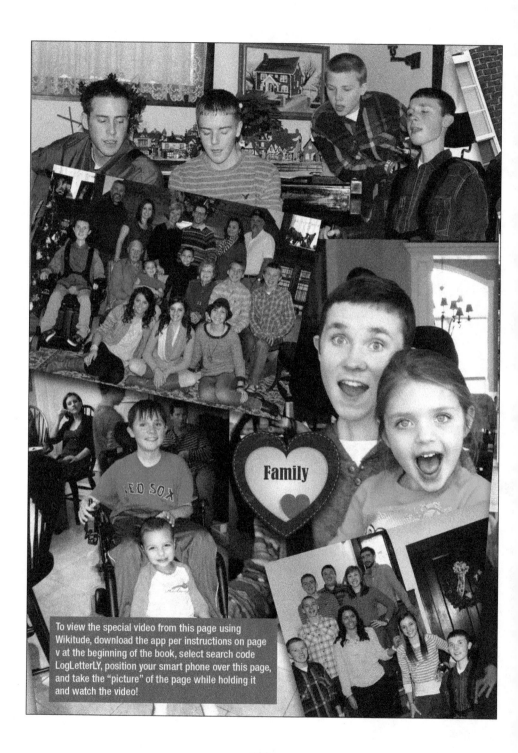

To view the special video from this page using Wikitude, download the app per instructions on page v at the beginning of the book, select search code LogLetterLY, position your smart phone over this page, and take the "picture" of the page while holding it and watch the video!

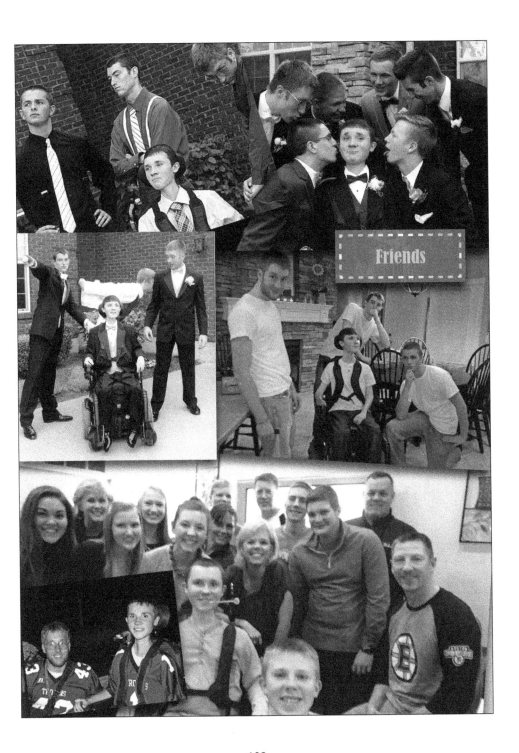

Friends

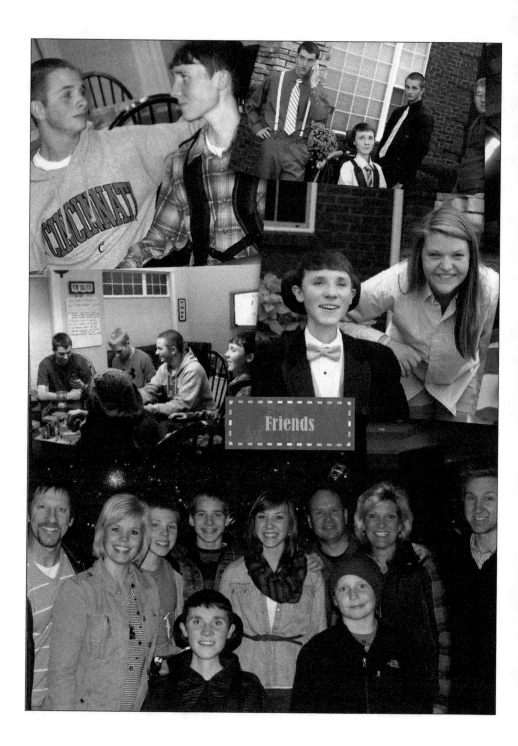

Friends

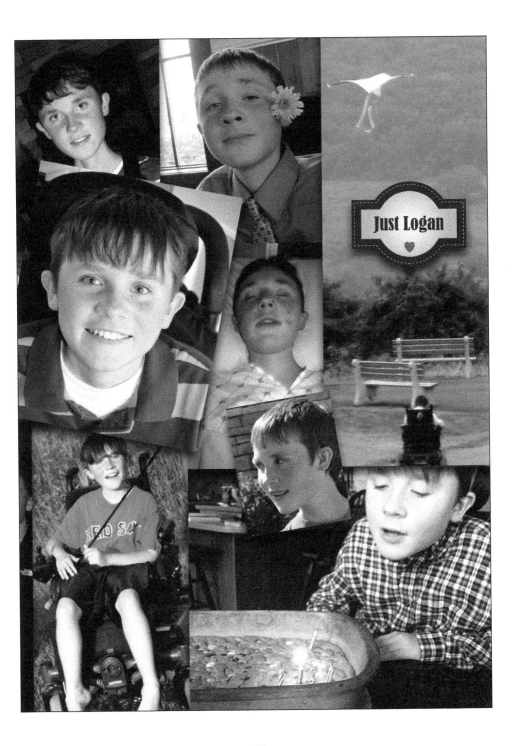

Just Logan

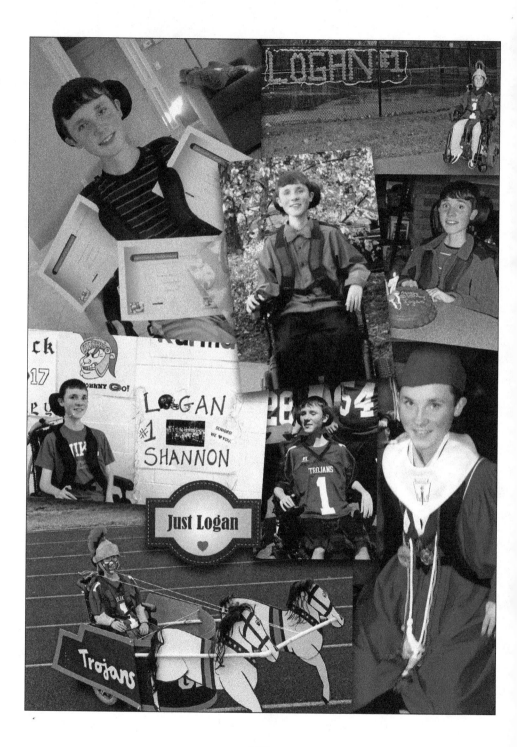

Chapter 16

Poem - "Logan, Life In The Chair"

A boy is born, and the family grows,
love is cuddled in soft baby clothes.
Logan is 2nd, and they all felt blessed,
not knowing the future, there'd come a test.
But over the years, tears would fall;
and giggles erupt about nothing at all.

Life is certainly a path unknown,
that makes us grip to a chaperone.
And who that is depends on where
we put our trust, our hope, our care.
Verses tell us of a hand that's sure,
powerful, tender and totally pure;
Who holds us during the life we've trod,
one who knows the Hand of God.

It took some time to notice a change,
Logan's walk was looking strange.
What was this, an innocent thing?
Or a deeper concern, an unsettling?
A closer look from the medical field,
a heartbreaking determination yield.

A serious sign, would come into play
that walking would stop, tough to say;
His uneven gate, for a child so young
would signal the start, not able to run.
Yet kids in his school, just didn't mind;
they'd help to support him, front and behind.
Accepted by all, he grew in that school,
There would be fights over Logan, that's cool.

His mind was still sharp, his body was weak,
His love was bold, but prognosis bleak.
Wheelchairs back then were pushed by hand,
Mom and Dad searched to at least understand.
Why it was now that this trial came?
They both held to God, no one to blame.
Questions abound, and hard to prepare;
This was their Logan, strapped in a chair.

But something was growing inside this young man,
That couldn't be known, supernatural plan.
Why would we think, that things must be bad,
When something like this can make us so sad?
A touch from the Lord, Almighty in ways,
Prepared him for duty, and so he obeys
The guidance from God, in prayer and in deeds.
That many are touched and Logan succeeds.
Befriending and guiding is who Logan is;
That leadership quality was naturally his.

Time went on and friend circles grew,
Something was special and everyone knew.
Logan's impact unfolded in hundreds of cases
Shows how hope responds in touching embraces.
For Logan's a man who is truly a man
With something to offer that few others can,

But in a way that's special and truly his own
Not just the surface but down to the bone.

His brothers and sister, his Mom and his Dad,
Invested in him, with all that they had.
Logan is part of his family, you know,
But they, too; are part of Logan as though
They're all knit together in a fabric of grace
Through every challenge that cannot replace

The love and respect that's grown over time
To watch Logan grow and his mountain to climb.
Together they gather, in love and in prayer,
Because way down the road, he won't need a chair.

Many've come forward to tell of how he
Has helped their character forming you see
Whose life is part of who they're become,
Invested in friendships to a real tidy sum.
And those who have known that he all along,
Was a friend and showed them how to be strong.

Logan can't run, or jump or play ball.
He also can't walk or stand straight and tall.
But Logan has something and handles with class
With those that he meets, friendships steadfast.

We all know some Logans who struggle with life.
It's not all their fault that they have such strife.
Sometimes we don't see what's right there in front
Where a person is waiting, to be perfectly blunt.
We miss who is there because we don't see
Past a condition that's pure irony;

We have them ourselves that others can tell
But we can't seem to perceive it ourself.
Logan's a man who likes love that is true.
It just doesn't matter with what he's been through
His life isn't over, he knows it's not "fair"
But he's exactly like us, except for the chair.

Chapter 17

More Loganisms and Thoughts

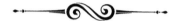

After Logan finished elementary school at Clough Pike (Pronounced "Cluff"), he went on to the Glen Este Middle School locally. It is part of the middle school / high school campus complex. Several elementary schools promote to that middle school, so when you read other school names, be advised that these were those schools.

Logan and I get into how he felt when students of other schools reacted differently than the students at the elementary school where they all knew Logan through all 5 years:

Lee: Now when you started at Glen Este Middle School, a lot of other kids began to show up from other schools like Brantner Elementary School, Willowville Elementary School, etc. These other kids did not have the benefit of seeing you during your school years at Clough Pike Elementary School. What was their impression of you when you started middle school?

Logan: They treated me a lot differently than the friends I had at Clough Elementary. I learned a lot about myself, by watching their reactions to me; and I learned a lot about them by my reactions to them. I didn't know people would treat me differently because I didn't see myself as different. I was just in a wheelchair. The acceptance of the other middle school kids took a couple of years. But most of them came around, and appreciated what I was going through. So as time went on, it got easier. One problem I had was that I tried to act like everything was no different. So I tried too hard sometimes to try not to be different, and to be more popular.

Another thing was there were a lot more students with all the other elementary schools now in one school. Basically I only knew about one third of the students in middle school. But in middle school, all the classes were arranged so that everybody got mixed; so I got experience with all the other students eventually. So other students from other elementary schools had to initially base how they knew me by how they saw me.

Lee: I remember high school very well, Logan. It was the worst eight years of my life (laughing with Logan)! I remember so many things from that experience vividly. I do not have a photographic memory or total recall. But I remember many things about that experience. I remember the people, the faculty, the administration, the building facility, the parking lot, the walks to and from school, some of the sports events, and especially the treatment of other students. I remember those who treated me right; and those who didn't... I was a radical introvert, and had very few friends. There were struggles at home and I found that escaping pain and withdrawing from everyone was part of the solution. In attempts to fit in, I didn't do too well.

For my junior prom, I didn't know what to do or who to ask. I even offered girls money to go with me; and they wouldn't accept the offer. I finally asked this one girl out and she said, "I'll go to the prom with you." She had been turning a few others down but agreed to go with me. She also said, "You are the first one to ask me since the accident." I laughed over the phone, and found out later she had a leg cast up to her hip. But she agreed to go to the junior prom with me. I took quite a ribbing from everybody for a number of reasons. The one that was obvious to me was how do you dance with the girl who has a leg cast on from her hip to her toes? It was quite an experience because everybody saw me as the guy who couldn't get a date with a girl who would be able to dance. The only one I could get was a girl nobody really wanted to take to the prom anymore.

So Logan, how did things go for you? Did you have a group of guys you hung around with? Did you have a girlfriend?

Logan: I had somewhat of a relationship in high school, but we could never go out in a traditional sense because she really wasn't allowed to. A casual meeting was okay, but wasn't allowed to seriously date until she was 18. Another issue was how do you really date a guy in a wheelchair, with the level of disability that I have? Too many times, most girls would think I was too cute, or too innocent to be considered as a boyfriend. I had to ask girls out, because they would not ask me. Sometimes it would really irritate me, because they would view me kind of as the same "cute" as they would their grandparents or some other older person confined to a wheelchair. It always bothered me. Sometimes they would be surprised when I asked them. That's a little bit of background of the issues I had with relationships back then.

The girl I was kind of going with back then decided she was going to go with someone else after a while. That decision really, really hurt, because I was so invested. It probably hurt more than it should have because I know, at times, I put too much of my identity into that relationship. She also went to a different school so that was part of the mix.

Part of the issue started back in middle school, when I began to have some anxiety attacks. I am not sure if it was related to the disease, the new school setting, or the fact that middle school

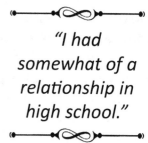

"I had somewhat of a relationship in high school."

"Too many times, most girls would think I was too cute, or too innocent to be considered as a boyfriend."

is where behaviors begin changing. I thought since I was having these beginning anxiety attacks, that everybody was having them in some way or another. This carried over into high school somewhat, but now I have settled into a much more understanding attitude since I've graduated.

But getting back to the "relationship"; when I was 17, I wanted to go with her when she was 15. I told her parents that I would wait until she was 18 if I could date her. And you know, I really started to like her. And again, after several months of being "together", she simply decided to start going out with someone else. But to this day, we remain good friends.

Lee: But in middle school, some of the relationships I've heard about don't even last one day. They agreed to go out with each other at first; and by the end of the day, they've broken up! Some miraculously last one week... In high school they tend to last a little bit longer, don't they? Even my granddaughter says that some kids in her class started going together at the beginning of the class, and then break up during that same class. In some relationships, they end because of something they saw that was tweeted, or that someone said something on Facebook, or something that someone texted to someone else. Or someone says, "I saw you talking to that girl, (or that guy) so I'm breaking up with you." (Both of us laughing)

Getting back to you, your grades were pretty good back then, weren't they?

Logan: Middle school, all A's. High school, all A's. In fact, all Shannons, all A's. My sister ahead of me was a valedictorian, I was a valedictorian, and my younger brother, Devon was a valedictorian. And my youngest brother, Corey, is also on his way to be a valedictorian when he graduates.

Lee: That's incredible. That's really incredible. Outstanding achievement. Logan, that's another book, don't you think?. (Both of us laughing) So after having a few prescriptions in middle school to address the anxiety you are having, did any of that change after going to high school? Did the prescription levels remain the same or were they revised?

Logan: I still have some anxiety issues, but the prescriptions have changed some over the years.

Lee: Are they related to the chair? Or are they related to the pressure of study? Or are they related to social interaction?

Logan: The anxiety issue came from different places, and sometimes it was worse than at other times. Sometimes just thinking and praying about it, and talking with my parents about it, allowed me to come to some conclusions. I had to try to figure something out on my own.

One of the issues that stemmed from the anxiety was a fear of speaking in front of other people. I was absolutely terrified to speak in front of people and it started in middle school. If I was asked to answer anything my face would get blood red and fear would grip me. And not only would my face get red but my chest would tighten up in almost a panic attack. But that would be the extreme reaction, and I thought every-body went through that. I thought that was normal and everybody went through that kind of nervousness. I didn't think I was different. Then I found out that others did not go through the nervousness like I did. I found out more and more it was just me. I just hated talking in front of people. And I knew I would have to speak when I gave a project report in school, and I would always feel anxiety coming on when it came time for the report to be given. As I think back in eighth grade, I don't know if I had that big of an issue back then. It was more anxiety in general not about speaking. But the speaking anxiety began growing once I got into high school. I used to get sweaty palms and my pulse used to quicken when I realized I had to answer something or explain something outside of normal conversation. And this was on top

"One of the issues that stemmed from the anxiety was a fear of speaking in front of other people."

of the disease and medical problems, the wheelchair issues, and maintaining good grades.

Lee: Do you think having this Duchenne Muscular Dystrophy has somehow helped you in school?

Logan: I don't know. And I really don't know, because I don't know what I might have been like without this disease. How does anybody really know how their life would have been if things had been different? Everything has been more difficult in most ways.

Lee: That's a pretty astute observation, Logan. It is a challenging thing to think about how your life could have been different, because we have no idea how any of our lives would've been different had circumstances changed; either with disease, with job relocation, with deaths in the family at different times, or with financial changes and challenges. I know God does enter into equations like these, and your story is special. I know your younger brother Devon played football and your youngest brother is involved in sports, too. Do you think you would've played football in high school?

Logan: Probably. Because of the love of the game of football my high school athletic department allowed me to be the team mascot, even in my wheelchair. (Laugh) I did not **intend** on being the mascot, and I didn't even **try** to be the mascot; but I was recommended by others and urged on by other players. I accepted the position of team mascot because I couldn't do what I really wanted to do, and that was play football. I ended up really enjoying it.

"Because of the love of the game of football, my athletic department allowed me to be the team mascot, even in my wheelchair."

Lee: Logan, I'd like to ask you something. God knows everything about everything all the time. There is nothing He **doesn't** know about. So we have to trust Him with all things, don't we? And God knows the future. God knows how good it could have been had not Adam and Eve goofed up. God knows every fact, every truth, and knows every circumstance about every person on the planet. He knows everything. I thought about this before and I wanted to ask you a question along that line. If you had played football in high school or even in middle school, God might have seen that you could have gotten seriously hurt or another circumstance could have happened going to a game, during the game, or coming home from the game, right? God could have seen ahead of time that there was tragedy if you were not involved in muscular dystrophy.

(Lee told a quick story about how the Lord directs things even when the people are non-believers). I worked for GE right out of college. I didn't know it but it was the only company that had a corporate presence in Louisville, KY of all the companies that came to the college campus for the open house.

When I got to Louisville, KY in an engineering job in the home appliance business, one of my first jobs in the kitchen range department was to reduce headcount by using automation. I started dating a lady in that building, and it was so funny that one of my first jobs was to eliminate that job she was working on. (Logan and I are both laughing). I ended up marrying her, and I never did get that job automated... God knew that my future wife was not in New England, but in Kentucky. You have to think about these things, and how God works in the lives of all people. He knows what He has to do to bring great glory to Him. And God knew about your life, Logan. There is no correct answer about how your life should have been, because if there was an answer, that's the way life would have gone. (Logan nodding in the affirmative) Your life is exactly the way it was supposed to be to bring God maximum glory. And Logan, you are impacting hundreds and hundreds of people through the life you are living now. (Logan nodding his head in affirmative again).

Logan, let me ask you another question. Do you know a man named ***Charles Krauthammer?*** He is on one of the cable news network channels. Charles was diving into a swimming pool when he was much younger and hit his head during the dive and became mostly paralyzed from the neck down, only allowing a few hand gestures. He was going to Harvard University and was in his early 20s when this happened, and now he is in his 60s and is a very accomplished commentator from the conservative viewpoint. Back when the injury happened, he thought about quitting college. He was actually convincing himself that because he was in a wheelchair, he was in no condition to finish.

Other people began to counsel him and told him not to give up. So he changed his mind and finished, and graduated in the top 1% of his class. He's a very brilliant man. Even though this man was confined to a wheelchair because of the physical injury and not a disease, it didn't change the fact that his mind was sharp. And I'm convinced Logan, that you and this book will have an impact for the Lord that will expand far beyond this community and region.

Logan: Yes, I think it will.

Lee: Everybody learns things from everybody, and I am certainly learning from you. (Logan smiles).

Chapter 18

Four More Friends Tell Their Stories

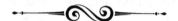

Four more friends share letters from the heart: Trevor Jones, Gabrielle Kirker, Nick Dierks, and Tim Berling all know Logan, and also offer their heart-felt affection for their friend, Logan Shannon.

Trevor Jones is one of Logan's closest friends going back to 2nd grade, and they've been next door neighbors for most of that time. Trevor reveals some of the joys and pains he experienced while growing up with Logan. He tells of how Logan, through coping with DMD, was an example of Christ's restoration in his own life.

Gabrielle (Gabby) Kirker has known Logan for years, and has grown closer and closer to him over the years. She goes to church with him, and she shares some thoughts about his humor, his faith, and his wisdom.

Nick Dierks has developed his friendship with Logan more recently. They, too, attend the same church together. He speaks about Logan's personal encouragement for him both in and out of military service in the Marine Corps.

Tim Berling has been such a close friend of Logan and his family, that he's practically family. He became close to the Shannons when he interned on staff at the church they all attended. He describes their friendship in terms of its "normalcy" despite the "differentness" others see.

First, Trevor Jones:

Dear Logan,

In hindsight the progression was obvious. And what progression was it? Our friendship, our growing up together, and our maturing into men. Do you remember the "technical" advantage our team had in playground kickball? Do you remember the episode of the stolen helicopter? Oh my, the memories.

What about the infamous cupcake adventure in the dead of night when we were in 5th grade? Talk about getting seriously busted!! I know you do! And then later as we were nearing high school age, I remember a stab in my heart that sent me into a rage like I've never felt before. My heart has now coped with that instant in time, Logan. I still have a hard time forgetting that feeling, as though it was yesterday.

(This picture on this page shows one of Logan's many bonding sessions, and friends who have contributed to this book. Logan is in the front center, Trevor Jones is the next one on the left on Logan's right hand, Joey Spiegel is at the far left at Trevor's right hand. Sam Becker giving Trevor a head lock, Macon Overcast is directly behind Logan, Logan's youngest brother, Corey is in the upper right. The only one not available for the book is Jeffery Benton, seated on Logan's left hand on the far right).

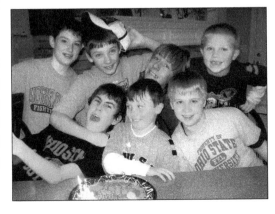

So let's go back in time to reminisce about those various times. First to those days in elementary school where "kickball stardom" was pretty straight forward for us. ***One wheel chair*** is all it took. I would kick and you would "run" faster than any of us mere-mortals could imagine. Obviously (known via the groans of our competitors at Clough Pike Elementary School) we were one killer team. No one could touch us!

A few years tick by. By this time, you and I were bonding as a team, sort of... I was the (ahem) trouble-maker; and you were the mastermind. One time I stayed over at your house and we came up with our greatest plan yet: during the deep night of your birthday, we would wait until everyone else went to sleep. Then we would carefully open the door trying to let it not make any noise, and slip silently through the darkness to where the collection of sweet baked stuff was. The goal was to steal some late night sweets and play with your new gadgets. So being the daring (foolish) kid I was, I listened to ***your*** urging and snuck out of the safe confines of your room to grab those goodies. I got what I could, and skillfully retreated back into the shadows. It seemed like our biggest success after I made it to the room unscathed and undetected. But it turned into a busting of a life-time. Your mom burst in just seconds into our celebration and caught us red handed, cupcake icing smeared all over our faces and a toy helicopter hovering mid-air. However, like true crim-inals, we remained side-by-side in our failure and punishment. (By the way, I still think of those days when I eat a cupcake!)

Skipping forward a few more years to the end of those dark years that are middle school. I think we were in 8th grade, and it was the close of a pretty normal day when we began our daily walk home after the school bell rang. The high school and the middle school were in the same campus and a few of the facili-ties were shared by both schools. The high school let out a little earlier than the middle school did, so taking our steps into the usually empty high school brought us into a situation I never could have imagined. I never expected what was about to happen! (I know you remember this). An unusual, but small group of freshman of clouded reputation, met us at the last set of interior doors of the last school hallway. Suddenly, a single comment from one of the guys' mouths in passing was followed by an unforgettable roar of laughter from the other two guys in the group. (There was also a girl in the group who didn't laugh and showed obvious distaste for that comment).

> *"I stopped and stared at them for a moment and finally caught up with you with a wounded heart and that word "cripple" echoing in my mind. We got to the exit doors going to the outside of the building and realized for the first time I saw Logan 'the kid in the wheelchair' and not who you really are."*

I stopped right there in my tracks with a lump in my throat, a deep pain in my heart, and fists clenched so hard my nails were about to break the skin in my palms. I've never been so close to fighting before; and yet, **you** kept "walking". I stopped and stared at them for a moment and finally caught up with you with a wounded heart and that word **"cripple"** echoing in my mind. We got to the exit doors going to the outside of the building, and for the <u>first time</u>, I saw Logan, "the kid in the wheelchair" and **not** who you really are. I knew you as "walking" before the wheelchair was required, so I never really embraced seeing you as anything else but "riding" in that wheelchair. Logan is my friend. He is not physically walking, but he is walking tall to me. So as I shook off that moment, I opened the doors to the outside and I noticed how strong you were and couldn't really understand why. You seemed to be above all those comments by those who just didn't understand. With tears gathering and making their way down from the corners of my eyes, no words were said as we both made it back to our houses. It hurt. It really hurt.

With hatred growing in my own heart for what they said and how they meant it, I saw you do something later that amazed me like nothing else had. Since **I** was angry, I told my mother, and she got ticked. The girl in the group must have also said something to some adults. Evidently, the pressure was put on that freshman from those sources over the next few weeks and he eventually uttered a somewhat forced apology to you. You looked right into his eyes and ***forgave that kid*** and accepted his apology! Incredible, simply incredible.

I would like to admit that I saw the progression by now, but I have to confess that I still missed it. As we continued our friendship into high school I saw your intelligence, strength, compassion, and joy in life and couldn't help but want it. I honestly felt a little selfish wanting the joy you had, after all that you had been through. It didn't take long after receiving Jesus Christ to see why I had envied you. You truly are a man who trusts that God is who He says He is, and that your sins have been paid in full by Christ our Lord.

The progression I was missing was

> *"...he eventually uttered a forced apology to you. You looked right into that kid's eyes and forgave that kid and accepted his apology. Incredible, simply incredible."*

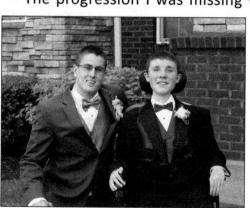

your growth in Christ. For you loved me so much that you decided to share your life with me, revealing Christ along the way. Logan, you carried me to the foot of the cross as I was too paralyzed in my sin to do it myself. Logan, I love you, man; and praise Jesus for all the work that He has done in you.

As we graduated, we both were among the group of 4 valedictorians, and I was proud to be with you as we closed out our high school days. You will always be my trusted friend. No matter how many times we get into cupcakes, get reckless with remote controlled devices, or have unkind things said to us by those who simply don't know better, I am proud to stand by you.

> **A Biblical example – Mark 2:3-5** *"And they came, bringing to Him a paralytic, carried by four men. And being unable to get to Him because of the crowd, they removed the roof above Him; and when they had dug an opening, they let down the pallet on which the paralytic was lying. And Jesus seeing their faith said to the paralytic, "My son, your sins are forgiven."* **(NASB)**

This is the scripture that reminds me most of Logan's role in my life. Logan is truly one of the men who carried <u>me</u> to Christ by how Logan loved me as a friend.

In His Grace,
Trevor Jones

From Gabrielle (Gabby) Kirker:

Logan Shannon is an extraordinary person, who happens to be in a wheelchair. I have known Logan for probably around 10 to 12 years of his 20-year life and in that time, our friendship has only gotten stronger and in the last year or so, we have grown really close.

One thing, among many things, that I admire about Logan is that no matter what struggle he faces with this type of Muscular Dystrophy, he never complains. I have never heard Logan complain about the struggles and trials he faces daily. Logan has this disease where his muscles have grown progressively weaker and weaker to the point that he can only move his fingers and above his shoulders, but he sees it as an opportunity to reach people who seem lost and without hope.

Logan has an enormous heart and passion for Jesus Christ and knows that a moral compass brings an inner peace and deep understanding of what is around us.

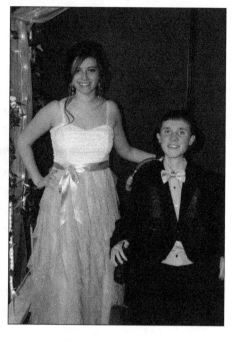

One funny thing that always sticks out in my mind about Logan is one time, when we were still in high school, a lot of the kids that went to our church would stand at my locker at the end of the day and chat. When we were all talking, a very loud and obnoxious group walked passed us and Logan said, "What would they do if I just sprang out my chair and karate chopped them all?" We all cracked up for at least 15 minutes.

Logan has more of a reason to be mad at the world and God than anyone, yet he turns that into passion and love.

Logan is an amazing friend and overall person and that is why I admire Logan Shannon. Logan is kind to everyone no matter how strange or ever rude that person is, Logan shows them love and has a heart for every one he encounters. Where to start on what Logan means to me.........

He inspires me every time I see him to be more like him because he strives to be more like Christ. Logan is the most hilarious and fun person I have ever met as well. Logan knows how to have a good time and always leaves me laughing at some hilarious joke he just told. I know that Logan is always there for me. If I have exams coming up or am nervous about something, Logan tells me he'll pray for me. He is a very encouraging friend!!

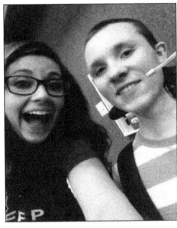

Two special times I remember about Logan: One is on our yearly church's mission trip to New York City, and the other is when he comes to a local college campus where I go and he leads a Bible study on Thursdays. In NYC, Logan was AMAZING! He had no hesitation about approaching people to witness to them for Christ or going on the subway, which was a huge struggle at times with his wheelchair and the adults trying to find subway train elevators that worked well or even worked at all. Logan would witness to everyone, probably more than some of the people on our Missions Team, including myself. He looked fearless and was just great there.

Logan knows his Bible and leads a Bible Study at my secular college every Thursday and I always benefit from it. He knows how to be approachable and to relate to people. Many people at my old high school and now my college have said, "Man, that guy is so nice and seems really cool. What is he really like?"

I have never had anything but amazing things to say about Logan. After people see me talking with Logan, realizing that we are friends, they always come up to me and ask me about him. One time, a totally random person saw me talking to Logan at The University of Cincinnati at Clermont where he leads the Bible Study and I could kind of see the guy staring. Logan left to go talk to someone else or leave or something (I can't quite remember that part). But when he left that person walked up to me and asked me why Logan is in a wheelchair. I told him his story about how he has Duchenne Muscular Dystrophy and that he can't move almost any part of his body, but that he is not angry or bitter about it and uses it to his advantage. The guy was so amazed and I told him how Logan is one of my greatest friends and he said this exactly, "That guy inspired me to be grateful for what I have and I didn't even talk to him." I admire Logan for his heart, his humor, and his love for people and Jesus.

Gabrielle (Gabby) Kirker

Now a quick communication from Nick Dierks:

Logan,

You have got to be the strongest and most spiritual person I've ever met to this day. You never skip a beat at being at church and you are always showing up to nearly every event that's scheduled. Also, you could definitely show me up when it comes to Bible verse memorization and your knowledge of the Bible. That's something to model after.

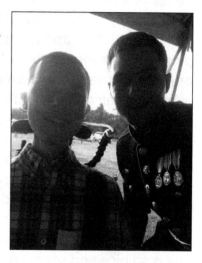

I remember getting to youth group on Wednesday and Sunday evenings and you would be one of the first people I would go up to and ask, "How are things going?" And no matter what, you had a smile on your face and always had something funny to say.

You are hands down, the nicest and easiest person to talk to any day of the week; and not to mention, you come from one of the sweetest families I know. Since I am serving in the United States Marine Corps, I'm always excited to see you when I visit home. I am glad I consider you a good friend. It's been good that I've gotten to know you through the years.

Nick Dierks USMC

Tim Berling writes his moving letter in a way that's cool. He writes it **directly to you** about his friend Logan.

I have thought about what to write in this letter about Logan for months. I started and stopped, and chewed on different ideas attempting to think about a signature moment, wanting to sum up who he is, or explain what he means to me with one story. After hours of contemplation, and months of thinking, it finally came to me: I **don't have** a signature moment with Logan, or a stand out story. The most amazing thing to me about Logan is

how normal and relatable he has always been, in light of literally crippling circumstances. He not only is just another one of the guys, **he just happens to be the best of us**. Muscular Dystrophy never conquered his mind, spirit, or soul. Rather, those different signature moments were like when we would pile him up in blankets so he could attend a chilly football game, or transform his wheel chair into a chariot to be the mascot at every Friday night football game. I watched him take forever to get 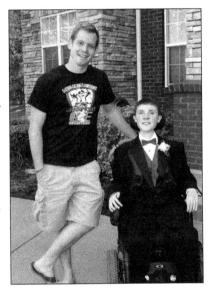 ready so he could look fresh and dapper, listened to him complain and joke about his particular pet peeves, sat around for hours watching TV shows, and talked and argued about our favorite sports teams.

At times, he was so completely comfortable and nonchalant about having Muscular Dystrophy that you forgot about it the way you forget a friend's hair color, or height. You know their hair color and whether they are short or tall, but it is so far in the background of your thoughts that it never comes up in conversation. Muscular Dystrophy not only didn't conquer Logan, he minimized his most obvious physical trait. He turned the first thing you see into inaudible background noise with a mischievous, but most extremely charming, and indomitable personality.

Those close to Logan know that it was neither easy, nor effortless. Like all of us, he had to become comfortable in his own skin. Of course, there were detours and road bumps along the way. We all have issues and problems, self-esteem issues or social anxiety from time to time. We are all different. But Logan's differentness (if that's a word), is on display for anyone and everyone to see. I always think how easy it would have been for Logan to just shut down and push everyone away, to wallow and drown in a pool of self-pity. He never did. He chose life; and he lives it abundantly, he lives it beautifully. I have watched him affect and influence thousands of people, seen him go through highs and lows, been with him when he laughed, and cried. He is, and will always be, just an extraordinarily normal friend.

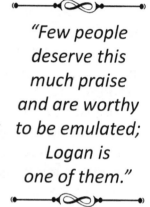

"Few people deserve this much praise and are worthy to be emulated; Logan is one of them."

Logan is a friend, confidant, peer, brother in Christ, and "family". He is everything everyone makes him out to be, and more. Biblical Scripture tells us to not brag, but to let others do it for us. Few people deserve this much praise and are worthy to be emulated, Logan is one of them. I am lucky to have him in my life, and forever thankful that God lead our paths to cross. In my mind's eye Logan isn't unlucky, disabled, or crippled, he is just an extraordinary person that does his best to love God and, to love others more than he loves himself. In his own weakness and frailty he found strength. He doesn't brag or complain, not that anyone would disagree. Logan is just Logan, wheeling around, smiling, laughing, and annoying me with his undying love for the New England Patriots. He has overcome more than most of us, yet he is just normal. He is however, the best normal anyone can ever be.

I love this guy!
Tim Berling

Chapter 19

Logan's Logic, Wit, and Daily Trials

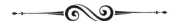

O ver the years, Logan has made brief comments and stated opinions about various issues and topics. I began compiling these with the intent of sharing them with readers who would like to peek a little deeper into Logan's insight, his light sarcasm, and sense of humor. So, I will list a few of many.

Also, we'll be sharing the preparation for a typical day. Logan doesn't just show up totally ready. When folks see him, he's already been through preparation with the total assistance of others. They physically take care of all the hygiene and handle the tasks behind the scenes. So the Shannon family was gracious enough to stage for me a mock "going to bed" and "getting out of bed" in the morning with Logan as the main event. It was astonishing to see so many steps that have to be done. It would be easy for us to take them for granted. These steps are done with precision, with process and with love.

First, let's look at Logan's wit, humor, and wavelength. After that, we'll settle back into participating with how Logan gets ready in the morning and how he gets ready at night.

- I try to use the voice of Morgan Freeman as my voice inside my head.

- Just realized that the little design on our toilet paper shows butterflies. I'm not so sure those butterflies appreciate what we've been using them for...
- I wore an I ♥ NY shirt today to jinx the Yankees and make the Red Sox win. Looks like it worked, I'm a genius!
- Raising your voice only makes you look insane.
- Awkward moments.... Hmmm (gotta love 'em).
- No pain, no pain.
- Love is Louder? How 'bout God's Love is Loudest !?!?
- So you like to chew? Maybe you should chew on my FIST!
- Hey! You really need to be revving it down.
- There is no charge for awesomeness, or attractiveness.
- Rockin' a fresh new 'do. Well, it's not that different than before, but it's still lookin' fresher.
- You can't be completely nuts, only like 3/4 nuts.
- TGIF... Thank Goodness I'm Fresh.
- I don't like to toot my horn, but ah-toots ma-goots!!
- You always gotta be watching out. Watching out for... *things...........*
- My Dad was trying to figure out Voldemort's name and this is what he said: Baltimort? Vandymore? Baldywart? Nose No More? hahaha good stuff.
- If I was Wendy, I would make sure I stayed away from Ronald McDonald. And quite frankly, she should avoid the Burger King too; no man with that much plastic on his face can be trusted.
- Here's a smile, if you're wearing argyle.
- The thing about pride is that the result always ends very badly. So my goal is/needs to be distancing myself from that attitude & behavior.
- Whenever your spirit gets low it only takes a second for grace to pick it back up to a higher place.
- I bet if I told you I can't independently itch my own mosquito bites you'd be able to restrain complaints really well. This is the struggle.

- I may or may not have recently spent some time working on my raptor sounds in preparation for Jurassic World. I don't know, you decide.
- The gospel of Jesus is a beautiful thing in that it truly is a message of warning wrapped in an even larger message of hope! Now that's cool.
- Leaning on God through the sacrifice of Christ translates to a continual demeanor of rest. Gotta admit that sounds pretty good, doesn't it?
- Drives past adult superstore:
  "Well that's a worthy cause... if we're talking about becoming an arsonist."

OK, now we need to rest our smiles a while as you join me in being part of Logan's day.

It should be noted that Logan's Mom, Tyra, helps Logan in the morning; and his Dad, Michael joins in the help at bedtime. This cooperative effort works pretty well, and is revised based on the respective schedules of Mom, Dad, and Logan's other family members. During the day, there are miscellaneous activities that can take place like friend visits, doctor's appointments, church attendance, music concerts and sports events that require Logan to be away from home. He is therefore relying completely on who he is with. It's fascinating! But let's concentrate......

Let's now get into the daily routine by dividing each day into two basic parts; the morning process and the evening process.

Typical morning process:

1) Turn off the sound monitoring system (for listening to Logan overnight) that was turned on the evening before.
2) Turn off bed controls, return bed to horizontal, and deflate all air bladder baffles lowering both ends and both sides to completely flat geometry.
   Keep in mind that Logan's bed is very complex.

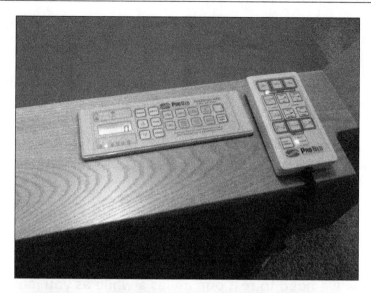

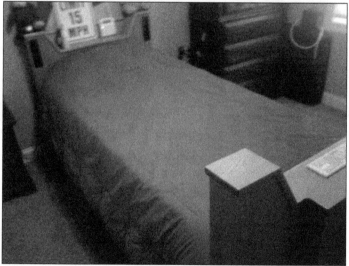

It has electronic controls and movements. There are many options for this type of bed, and individual needs and budgets will determine which level is required. (Logan's bed is the Freedom Bed by ProBed)

3) Turn off bi-pap machine hook-up
   Remove air manifold mask from Logan's face.
   Clean and store unit, hoses, and mask away in room.

4) Remove specific geometrically shaped pillows from under his legs, reshape and store away.
Remove bed covers and store away.

5) Pick Logan up physically, carry him to the bathroom and place him in a special water-proof PVC pipe-type chair structure and seat assembly which supports him over the toilet first. Toilet use is by gravity only due to Duchenne Muscular Dystrophy. This requires various periods of time which may be different each occasion. After that, Logan is wheeled into the shower area. The shower area threshold has been removed down to floor level so the PVC chair rolls easily into the shower area. After washing his hair and body, he is toweled dry and wheeled out in front of the mirror and sink. Here he is shaved, deodorant and lotion is applied, hair is combed, teeth are brushed, and he's ready to be dressed.

6) When Logan attended school, he had to get up at 5:00 AM to proceed through all the steps to be ready for class by the 7:15 AM start of classes.

7) When Logan is wheeled back into his bedroom, he is lifted out of the special bathroom seat assembly and placed on the bed again. He picks out his clothes and he is always dressed for the right occasion. This is an ***all-verbal effort*** here. The clothes have to be coordinated for the occasion. After dressing and getting everything right (like tucking, fitting, belt fit, and shoe tightness), Logan is lifted off the bed, put into his wheelchair, and strapped in for the day's activities.

8) Certain adjustments for his "comfortability" can take varying amounts of time and effort, typically from 10 to 30 minutes. The seat cushion on the wheelchair is made of multiple air chambers that need to contour to Logan's body.

9) Logan's breakfast is determined by dietary guidelines and personal preferences.

10) Lunch varies depending on whatever the day schedule is, and where.

Logan may request stretching, scratching, arm placement, etc., during the day; and family and friends assist however they can.

Typical evening process (similar to morning except extra steps):

1) Cough assist machine – Do as needed daily; more often if doctor recommends; and more often if congestion is present. - Machine simulates coughing by forcing air in and then pulls it out fast. This duplicates a cough, and removes mucus and phlegm, if any. If phlegm is present, then he spits into a cup for disposal.

2) Bi-pap machine hook-up:
   - Fill a small reservoir with water for vapor.
   - Use only when it's time for bed, and in reclining position.
   - Air manifold attaches to head, and locates over nostrils. It takes time to locate precisely, with exacting adjustments. Operates all night with programmed regularity.

3) Once in bed, specific geometrically shaped pillows are arranged for maximum comfort.
   - Logan's knees can't bend, but hips can rotate
   - Special soft memory Z-flo foam pillows are placed under knees. There can be much time spent getting exact final positioning.
   Blankets are placed on Logan.

4) The special, complex and programmable Freedom Bed by ProBed is in Logan's room.
   - Precise positioning is built in for maximum comfort.
   - Head / torso can be lifted as separate function.
   - Knees can be lifted as a separate function.
   - Built in air bladder baffles exist all along the edges of the bed for creating a soft side fence on both sides of the bed.

There are also baffles at each end of the bed that can elevate his head or his feet independently.

Then the bed is programmed for "rotating" Logan during the night. (This prevents bed sores, and keeps circulation at optimum)

On the bed's current settings, from horizontal, it can swing up to 30° each direction. Bed goes from horizontal to up to 30° to the right and stays. Bed returns to horizontal after 15 to 30 minutes (adjustable). It swings to up to 30° in the other direction. The bed returns to horizontal after 15 to 30 minutes. This cycle repeats all night until turned off.

The side bladder baffles stay inflated all night so Logan doesn't roll out of the bed during rotation.

5) The sound monitoring system is turned on so Mom and Dad can hear either Logan or any unusual sounds during the nighttime hours.

So now it's more clear as to all the things necessary for Logan to be ready for events, trips, dining out, or to work on this book. The support team is so important when it comes to the success of those who need assistance.

During his younger years, there were times of injuries due to different reasons, but a primary one was simply because of the transition from full muscle control to the beginning of the decline. So, when Logan would participate in physical activities, his mind would tell his legs to respond the way they used to. But when they didn't, the leg would occasionally be off the exact position and would sustain an injury. Other times, other crazy circumstances would happen that resulted in fractures. We have all experienced our own or our family members who have had broken bones from random circumstances.

Logan has had several casts and braces over his early years to help him through those times of healing. You will see pictures of those casts and braces and what happened during those specific times.

<u>Blue cast</u>: Was put on when the family's first dog, a Siberian Husky; got the leash wrapped around his foot. The dog was excited over something and the combined forces from the leash and the subsequent fall broke Logan's foot. It was a cast that went up to mid-thigh to upper thigh.

<u>Medium green cast</u>: Was when Logan was running later on and accidently stepped into a depression where an old water main ditch was and the dirt had settled in his yard. The awkwardness of his body position made him fall and he broke the same foot. It was a cast that went up to just over the knee.

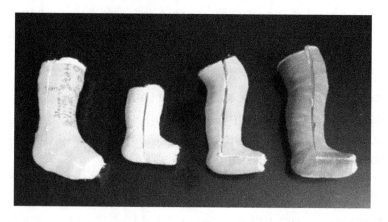

<u>Yellow cast</u>: Was just after Logan got out of his medium green cast, he fell again in an awkward position, and re-broke it. This time the cast only was a calf cast, not going up to the knee.

<u>Lime green cast</u>: Was when Logan and his brothers were wrestling on the couch. Logan was in 4th grade by this time, and when his brother, Corey, jumped off the couch onto Logan's ankle, it broke the foot again. This was a cast that went up to his knee. This was the last cast Logan had to wear.

Logan also wore leg braces for assistance in daily activities and for rest. These began during 2nd grade and went through 7th grade where they became too painful to wear. They were being used over time to simply postpone the inevitable. Some braces were full leg braces and some were just lower leg braces. As the disease progressed, his feet began turning downward and inward slightly at the ankles. The braces not only helped Logan to walk for longer periods of time, but the foot portion also provided a support that kept Logan's foot in straighter alignment with his lower leg.

<u>Purple braces</u>: The full leg brace was worn during the day doing daily activities including walking. The foot brace was worn during night time hours while sleeping. These braces began being worn in 4th grade.

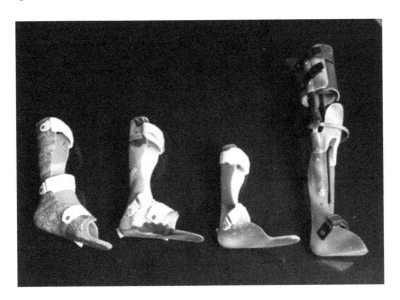

<u>The pinkish / buff color brace</u>: Was the next one to be worn at night. It was larger due to the growth of Logan's leg.

<u>Blue brace</u>: Was worn through 7th grade at night to continue the supporting and straightening functions. This was the last brace Logan wore because the gradual inward turning of his feet was not being slowed. The pain became too much.

The full time use of a powered wheelchair began before the discontinued use of the braces, and became a constant companion for Logan. As the years went by, he would transition from adolescent wheelchairs to a full-sized adult powered wheelchair.

As we look at the mechanical assistance over the years, Logan's personality, thoughtful spirit, wisdom, and coping skills were also being honed and developed. It can be said that as his physical body was in decline, his mind and heart was ramping up. His strength of will was deepening, and his realization of a greater calling was becoming more evident.

What is Logan's ultimate purpose in life? What is he supposed to do? How is he being prepared for a greater service than he expected? How has his family grown?

The answers to these questions may never be realized until the book closes on this world. But one thing can be assured: Logan will be faithful, his family and his friends will continue their support, and the example of his endurance, his insight, and his faith will affect countless people who cross his path.

It's time to read more about Logan and his life.....

Chapter 20

Three More Friends Tell About Logan

Three more friends share letters from the heart: Morgan Gibson Bailey, Jordan Large, and Kamen Powell. They have all known Logan, and bring their own personal feelings to you about their friend.

Morgan Gibson Bailey has been a friend of Logan's basically their whole lives. She recalls when they were prom prince and princess together and tells of how she would regularly visit him as he recovered from scoliosis surgery. She admires Logan for his God-born endurance with his difficulties.

Jordan Large graduated with Devon (Logan's younger brother) and has been a good friend of Logan's for years. In her letter, she explains how Logan's joy and encouragement have always been a blessing. She sums it all up by recounting the night they went to prom together.

Kamen Powell and Logan are life-long friends. As far as childhood friends go, they were the closest. For his contribution, he chose to include an essay he wrote while at West Point. In the essay, he expounded on what "selfless service" means through his interactions with Logan.

First, Morgan Gibson Bailey:

Dear Logan,

Where do I begin? I've known you ever since I was born (but of course you always make sure you remind me that you are older... by just two months). We have shared so many great memories together through the years. One memory that stands out to me was our junior year of high school when you won prom prince and I won prom princess. That could not have been more perfect; our parents were so proud. I remember the Sunday morning after that prom when we went into church

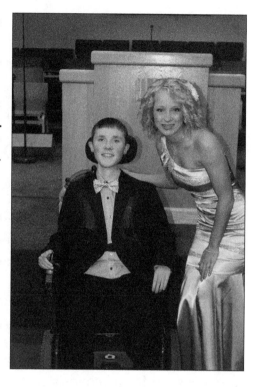

and everyone in our youth group referred to us as "prince" and "princess". The younger teens at church always looked up to you as a strong Christian individual. You lead study groups and sang in our youth praise team during Wednesday night church.

Other memories in high school include the summer of our sophomore year when you had a major back surgery and I came and saw you every chance I had. I was on the school tennis team and I remember walking to your house after practice since you lived close to our high school, and I would bring you gifts or specially baked treats. I would just spend time with you since you were not able to go anywhere over your long recovery period. The following summer we went on a mission trip together to New York City. It was amazing to be able to have the opportunity to share the gospel with the people there and see so many saved by receiving Christ as their personal Savior. While we were there we learned that New York was not made to always be handicap accessible. Finding the subway entrances that had elevators wasn't always easy, especially when they only worked half the time. Even with all the complexities trying to get around, you always made the best of the situation. We take so much for granted!

Speaking of what it takes to make the best out of a situation, you are an amazing example of exactly that. Many people do not realize how well they have it. They often come up with the flimsiest excuses of why they can't do things. You **have not chosen** to let your disability get in the way of your life and you **have chosen** to let God have complete control. You have truly given meaning to the verse "With men this is impossible; but with God all things are possible." Matthew 19:26. You have never used your disability as an excuse for anything, although you have used it to reach out to others and share 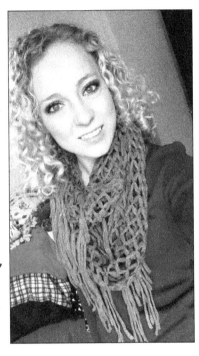 what God is doing for you in your life. Yes, you need help with a lot of specific things, but that does not stop you from living your life to the fullest. God has the master plan for each of our lives, and yours is no exception.

You and I have always been close friends, and you have been a great encouragement to me in many ways in my life as well as my walk with God. I know I am not the only one you have been an encouragement to. You were the valedictorian of our high school class of 2013. You gave a speech where you shared the reason for your success. You spoke on God's role in your life and how He is the only way to heaven. Your speech was given at our graduation ceremony in front of our whole senior class, their friends and families. God used you in an amazing way that day and throughout your high school career. Even now that we are out of high school and growing up, you are still an amazing friend and accountability partner. I feel that one of the reasons our friendship is so close is due to our shared love of God. We grew up in the same church (where we still attend regularly), and now have a Bible study together once a week outside of church with a group of our mutual friends. Having you as a friend is very important to me and I am truly blessed that God has given us this friendship.

Love, your friend,
Morgan Gibson Bailey

And now Jordan Large gets her chance!

Dear Logan,

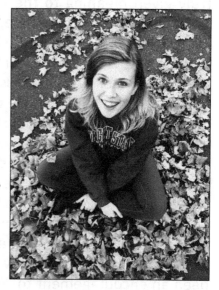

How do you create a letter that authentically communicates the blessing that is **you**? Your joy influenced the halls of our high school unlike anything else I've ever seen, and for so many people, *you have already been the author of some of the most beautiful memories*. You know, this letter has been difficult for me to write. I spent a lot of nights looking at an empty computer screen because I wasn't exactly sure how it was possible to put into words the way you have impacted my life; the way you challenged me, encouraged me, and blessed me. You are the kind of person anyone can take one look at and know that you love God unconditionally; simply because of the joy that radiates from you despite the trials you face.

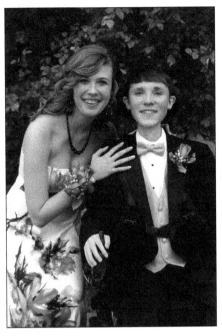

You have always been the kind of person who truly notices people, and the kind of person whose words could make hearts ache a little less. And how can someone "author a special memory"? You did! And it was prom night....... What you may not have known about that night, was how much it truly meant to me. Every girl dreams of the perfect high school prom and you certainly gave that to me. From your creative invitation, to picking out your tux, to watching you be crowned prom prince; it was spectacular! And I'm not sure if I've ever really gotten to truly thank you for it all. We were an unconventional couple and had to do things a little differently than everyone else, but I wouldn't change a thing. It was a night of blessed conversation and sweet, sweet friendship— which is more than I could ever ask for.

Love,
Jordan Large

Kamen Powell definitely wanted to contribute with this:

First of all, after requesting a letter several weeks previous to his reply, Kamen sent me Logan's letter with this explanation:

Hey Lee,

Thank you for your incredible patience with me. I finally now have the time to send this to you. I have been awfully busy with my school work here at West Point.

I hope this essay that I wrote last year at the United States Military Academy Preparatory School helps and is a big contribution to Logan's book.

In short, the prompt of this essay was to write a narrative story in which you learned a valuable lesson through a real-life experience. This experience I had with Logan truly showed me the kind of person I want to strive to be: *A person of selfless service*. With this experience, and many others I have had with helping others through mission trips and other events, I have learned to put others before myself. I believe this characteristic has gotten me to the place I am now.

Have a blessed evening.
Very Respectfully,
Kamen Powell

Lee, here is my essay, to use as my "letter" for Logan's book:

When I was 6 years old, I made the biggest transition of my life. Because of my father's job, our family was to move from Fort Lauderdale, Florida to Cincinnati, Ohio. At this time of my life, I was familiar with palm trees, beautiful beaches, and Walt Disney World. Moving to such a far and unfamiliar place made me nervous. I didn't know what to expect. Would I be able to get along with my peers? Would they accept me? Would I be able to make new friends? These questions and many others constantly floated through my head. I was unsure of what my future would be like. But surprisingly enough, all of these questions were answered within seconds of pulling into the driveway of our new home.

The moment our family stepped out of the car, our new neighbors, not only adults, but a number of kids about the same age as my brother and me, came up to us and welcomed us with open arms. The kids asked if we wanted to play with them.

Immediately, my brother and I hopped out of the car and began to play hide and seek with them.

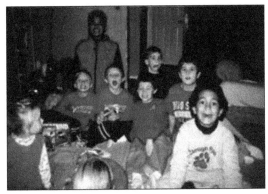

During our time playing with them, we got to know each one of the kids in the cul-de-sac. But there was one that was different from the rest. He was a member of the Shannon family. As we played hide and seek, I noticed he ***couldn't run as fast*** as everyone else. I could tell his running was something he could not control. So I asked his brother, Devon Shannon, what was wrong with his older brother, Logan. Devon explained that his older brother had a thing called Muscular Dystrophy.

(Shown above is a picture of Logan and his friends. Kamen and his brother, Hunter; plus Logan's brother Devon and others.)

After hide and seek, I went into the house and navigated my way through the maze of moving boxes and all our furniture temporarily placed in different parts of the house. I approached my dad and asked him, "Hey Dad, do you know what Muscular Dystrophy is?" He looked at me with a puzzled face and responded, "Yeah, why do you ask?" So I told him one of the kids that I played with had it. At the time, I didn't understand the significance of it, and I could tell my father was in shock by the news he had just heard.

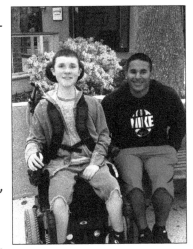

He told me that Muscular Dystrophy was a rare disease that weakens the muscles of the body and significantly affects one's ability to perform physical activity. After my father was finished explaining, I made the decision to do whatever I could to help Logan. When the first day of school arrived, I was fortunate to be in the same class as him. Every opportunity I had to help Logan, I took it. As the year went on, we became close friends.

One day, Logan's family asked us to go to church with them. We were looking for a church to go to anyway and we took them up on their offer and went to their church the next day. There were several activities for kids at the church that day like races and different competitions. I decided to enter a race because I like competing and winning. I saw that my friend, Logan, also entered the same race, and wished him the best of luck. I was on the line ready to take off. I looked to my left and to my right and was determined to get the title of first place in that race. The race was to see who could go from one end of the church basketball court to the other end the fastest.

The announcer took his place at the starting line and made sure everyone was lined up and no one was ahead of the other on the line. When everything was set, the announcer yelled in a loud voice, "Ready, set, GO!!" I roared off the line at full speed ahead, and the other end of the court got closer and closer. I was leading the pack and I was determined to show everyone that I was the fastest. But half-way down the court, I thought, "What about my new friend? How's he doing?" I turned around for just a moment and saw him really struggling to run. I could tell he was giving it all he could but couldn't keep up with the rest of the kids because of that thing called Muscular Dystrophy. So I had a BIG decision to make.....

Should I finish in first place and help him afterward?
OR
Should I give up my chance at first place and turn around
and finish **WITH** Logan?

I never regretted the decision I made; I stopped just short of the finish line with all the other kids right behind me nearly running into me. It was like I was in a theme park, moving from side to side, as if I was trying to find my mom or dad. So, I turned around and went back for Logan. I had to dodge several other kids to keep from getting knocked over, but I got to him quickly. I had him hop on my shoulders and we finished the race TOGETHER!

That event fortified our relationship from that moment onward. And as time went on, his symptoms gradually got worse and worse. He soon was in a push-type wheelchair and unable to walk. Whenever I was with him, I was the one who pushed him in the wheelchair and tended to whatever he needed, as long as I was at his side. I continued to assist him until I moved back to Florida four years later. To this day, I still stay in contact with him, and our families see each other at least once a year. Logan and his family still live in Cincinnati, Ohio.

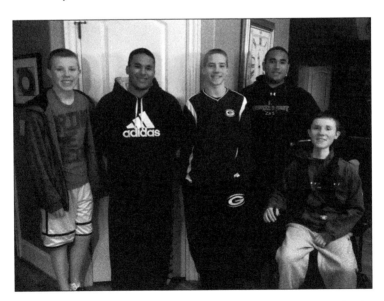

The moment that I made the decision to not finish the race and to carry Logan on my back, to cross that finish line together, has made me the person I am today. On that day, I truly learned what it meant to put others before myself. It is a virtue that I live by every day. I have also been able to help many others through mission trips and other special events.

I believe the biggest reason I came to West Point is to serve others as an Army officer and to continue to live by Army values that all soldiers strive for: ***Selfless Service.***

Kamen Powell

Shown on the previous page are all three Shannon brothers and the two Powell brothers.

Chapter 21

Logan's Valedictorian Speech and Message to a Church Group

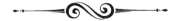

- Logan's Valedictorian Speech at graduation.
- Logan's Message on prayer at a youth Bible study.
- Logan shares his faith as he wrote to Mark Cahill.

Logan was one of the valedictorian speakers at his graduation, which was recorded on video and can be watched using the Wikitude **app over** the next full page w/ code (LogLetterHSG).

This book contains a **great video play feature** hidden in this chapter. Wikitude allows a reader to position a smart phone over designated pages, take the "picture" of the page while holding it, and watch a prepared video directly from that page. Review directions to watch the video at the beginning of the book on page viii.

The text from this speech is below. The text from his spiritual message on prayer follows the graduation speech. It was also recorded on video and can be watched using the same app.

The first section on the graduation speech video with all speakers is 14:20 (14 minutes and 20 seconds) long, and Logan speaks from the 8:00 mark to about the 10:45 mark.

At the graduation, Macon Overcast speaks first, then Molly Ballitch, then Jake Velten, then Logan, then Trevor Jones.

Logan makes his way to the front of the stage where the floor stand microphone is located. Macon Overcast holds the written text for Logan as he begins his address:

"Alrighty! For me to make the next few minutes about anything other than what I'm about to; would be to me, empty and almost meaningless. And what I want to make them about is the relationship I have with my Lord and Savior, Jesus Christ. (cheers)

It's who I believe in and it's what I believe in, and it's what makes me who I am. So, if you're here tonight, thinking it's impressive that I've made it to being one of the valedictorians amidst all of my struggles and my circumstance of having Muscular Dystrophy, let me stop you right there. Because without Jesus in my life, there's no way I would have been able to do what's been done at all. In fact, I'd be a completely different person, and very possibly miserable all the time.

And I'll be the first to admit that there are times I do get discouraged by my life and want to give up. But I never do, because of the one thing that keeps me going. And that's Jesus. All thanks to Him. Plain and simple, there's no way around it. Everything I've ever accomplished, I've done through Christ, and for Christ. That's all there is to it. It's all because of Him, and not because of me. The song, **Total Praise** says it best, *"He is the source of my strength, He is the strength of my life, and that is my anthem of praise to Him."* So again, this has all been in and to the Name of Jesus. I have to give Him all the glory for this one.

My point in sharing this is that if there's any advice I could ever give it would have to be linked with Jesus in some way.

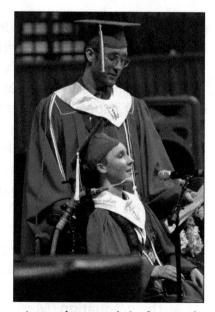

Logan's speech in front of his graduating class.

And the advice I have tonight is that, we're all going to face unexpected and difficult periods in life.

It's been pretty tough for us up to this point, and through this past year; and college life will have its hard times, too. Beyond that, everyone in this room will face financial difficulty, the loss of a loved one, an illness that shakes their world, some relationship problems they can't seem to get past, at some point in their life. And in the middle of those struggles, you will turn to a million different things in order to solve the problem, but most of those things just don't help at all.

And whether you believe me or not, there is only ONE THING that you can turn to, that will truly set you free from the struggle; and it's Jesus Christ. I promise that the hope and love that can be found in Him will free, fill, and sustain you.

So, if you ever find yourself in a situation like the ones I just described, my belief is the best thing we can ever do is to turn to God through Jesus. And that's what you should do, because He wants you to and He loves you. After all, He died on the cross for you. And that's all I have to say. So thank you! (cheers followed by standing ovation, including **everyone** on the stage)

Trevor Jones speaks after Logan and announces he is also a follower of Jesus Christ.

———◦———

Logan's message about prayer is next. Logan asked me back then if I would come visit in the teen room at the church we both go to, and listen to his message to the teens (He had just graduated from Glen Este High School, so he knew most everyone there anyway).

I sat with Logan's parents and assumed the attitude of the older, wiser senior figure with experience in spiritual maturity. I didn't have the disposition of being better than Logan, but I erroneously embraced the fact that I was there to review his message, and not necessarily learn from it. But the Lord essentially took me to the woodshed as Logan brought forth a powerful challenge showing me that any person in the hands of the Lord, deserves to be listened to. At the conclusion to that lesson, I wrote about my experience listening to God directing Logan through a vital lesson on the topic of prayer. Here's what I wrote:

> "After a brief introduction, a faint whirring sound could be heard as the motorized wheelchair made its way up the access ramp to the platform. There was no procession. There was no fanfare. There was no pretense. There was just the presence of a young man who felt deeply in his heart to share something very important to an audience of attentive young people and some adults. This high school valedictorian did, in fact share his heart. His name is Logan Shannon………

> Yet, the radiant, smiling face of that young man who is experiencing the ravages of Duchenne Muscular Dystrophy from a very young age seemed determined to minimize the issue of the wheelchair. He had been in one so long that it was second nature to him, so they functioned as one. When Logan began to speak, electronic devices in the crowd grew silent, normally restless teenagers became still, and a hush fell over everyone. We could tell this was not going to be a time of "same old, same old". The preparation, prayer, and research done were evident.

> Logan maneuvered his wheelchair back and forth across the platform effortlessly, bringing the message of the importance of PRAYER in our daily lives. His humor and honesty came through, disarming skeptical minds about his capability of delivering

his thoughts at this high of a competency level. With his lung capacity well below 20% of normal, he had to take occasional inhales from an oxygen tube leading from equipment that was contained in the wheelchair. This way, he was able to maintain the flow and content of his topic. He even coped with a surprise glitch with the new model wheelchair with humor and grace.

As I think back over the years, many who had grown up with Logan and his family thought many things and had so many questions. We had seen him with the initial stages where his walking was uneven, then with required use of assistance. Finally, a wheelchair was implemented. We all watched him remain as active as he could with the joy stick features of those first wheelchairs. But as the disease progressed, he gradually grew weaker and weaker. So the strength necessary to just move the joy stick had to be considered.

Back to the present again, where Logan was reading from prepared notes positioned on strategically placed music stands on the platform. There was hardly any movement in the room, and each one of us was compelled to deal with each bullet-point of that topic. When he finished his moving and heart-felt message, there was immediate applause. He guided the wheelchair skillfully back down the ramp and over to a place in the back.

This was no ordinary moment in time. This was no ordinary event in the lives of everyone who listened. The topic was from the timeless wisdom and power of the Holy Bible and he delivered flawlessly. Even with less than 20% lung capacity, Logan Shannon breathed out a riveting exposition of the Lord's Prayer. He touched lives because he allowed Jesus Christ to be the center of it all. He was a blessing because of the deep truths that were explained simply and concisely. He urged us to take prayer seriously because God takes it seriously. He urged us to read the Lord's Prayer seriously because Christ shared it seriously.

I have been a Christian for over 40 years and have been out of high school for over 45 years. I have been a substitute teacher for Biblical studies and have been asked by some churches to bring the main message on Sunday mornings, so I know what preparation means. But when that high school valedictorian allowed Almighty God to talk through him, it became obvious that God will use whomever He wants. And for this session, I was taken back to school......."

The following few pages contain the first section of Logan's text from that Wednesday evening, September 25, 2013, challenge to the teens at our church.

Devon Shannon, the younger brother of Logan, assisted in Logan's documentation on the music stands assembled on the platform.

"All right. So, we're going to be talking about prayer tonight. And really, me and Pastor Bob (Bob Johnson – Youth Pastor at First Baptist Church of Glen Este) didn't do that on purpose. It kind of happened this way, where I came to him and told him I had a message on prayer I've been working on. And it's been something that kind of was laid on my heart; I'm going to say it was back in like February (2013) and has slowly grown into something.

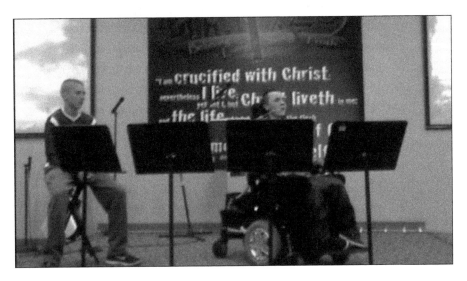

(Watch video of Logan's lesson by hovering phone over this full page and engaging the free **Wikitude** app with search code labeled LogLetterYM)

So it's just kind of cool how that lined up with today being "Prayer at the Pole" which we didn't really plan that. So anyways, this was laid on my heart a while ago. And lately with what has been laid on my heart, God has been rejuvenating my prayer life. And my hope is that all that I have planned tonight is going to kind of rejuvenate *your* prayer life, too; to give you insights on ways to just really tap into the power of prayer.

A lot has happened in my life so my purpose in taking a break off from school this year, (and not going to college and stuff) was to grow closer to God and so this has just lined up perfectly.

I find myself wishing that while I was in middle school and high school, that I had prayed a lot more than I had. And it's really changed my life. I'm sorry that this isn't really a message on the power of prayer, but it's more on the **way** to pray. And what it says in Matthew 6 is important, so you want to go there now. And the reason this isn't a message of an ordinary topic, I think we all understand that prayer is extremely powerful. And this is more about the way to pray by sharing practical tools and techniques; how to pray by looking at the way Jesus did as our example. So we're going to be running through **The Lord's Prayer** to do that. And before that I wanted to give you <u>four points</u> before the message.

<u>The first one</u> that I have is that when we don't pray, the Devil wins the battle. And I kind of got this because this passage is on page 666 in my Bible, and when I first came across it, I was like, 'Oh shoot!', I don't know if I need to be preaching this. I'm on some dangerous ground knowing that. But that thought was completely ridiculous. No, that's completely ridiculous. So, God was the guiding power in that. Satan absolutely trembles when we pray. And he loves it when we don't pray. And he will stop at nothing to get us not to pray. So, I need you guys to understand that. The devil understands how powerful prayer is, so we need to, too. We need to remember he wants to keep us from praying and digging into what personal conversation God wants to have with you.

<u>And my second point</u>, before I get started is that the Bible tells us to pray without ceasing. That's

somewhere in First Thessalonians which I didn't realize, but "PB" (Pastor Bob) told me that this was one of you guys's verses to memorize on the little list for this year. So that was kind of cool. But, so basically, that's just saying pray about anything and everything that comes to your mind.

And the third point kind of goes right alongside with that. In Psalms, David tells us to have a praise continually on our lips; to constantly be thanking Him for whichever things He lays on our heart. And these two ideas are married in the verse Philippians 4:6, "Be anxious for nothing, but in everything by prayer and supplication, with thanksgiving; let your requests be made known to God." So, pretty much bring all your requests and let all your praise be made known unto God.

And the last point is to pray **out loud**. Whenever we find Jesus praying in the Bible, we see that He is speaking it out loud, rather than silently doing it in His mind. And I've just found this additional thing is so much more powerful about praying out loud. It makes God's presence so much more tangible and so much more real, and I know it will for you guys, too. Because seriously, I've been doing this more than I ever have in the last couple of months, and I just know that God's presence is real when I pray out loud.

Also, the forces of darkness tremble at a spoken prayer because I understand that in those moments, the power of Jesus is flowing there and in you. The reason is because the demons and the Devil cannot, **they can't** read your thoughts the way that God can; they can only hear what you're **saying**. And when they hear you praying to God, they know you're relying on Him and not on yourself. When you start praying out loud, you can, at times, have the "I feel weird" moments. You can still pray silently, but whenever you can, stay with praying out loud. There's actually another thing, another little thing that came into my mind as I was coming here, that a lot of times, we look at prayer as one of the hardest disciplines of our Christian life. I think we need to bring ourselves to the point where it's **not** a discipline; it's something we just enjoy doing.

Jesus is truly our best friend, and we enjoy spending time with the Creator of the universe that loves us....... so much. And when we do that, it will change our attitude about a lot of things.

Logan completes his opening statements, and asks Devon to do final arrangements of his notes on the music stands.

Before I get into the actual passage I want to give you guys a little background for what's going on with **The Lord's Prayer**. So I'm going to read Matthew 4:23 through 5:2. 'And Jesus went about all Galilee, teaching in their synagogues, preaching the gospel of the kingdom, and healing all kinds of sickness and all kinds of disease among the people. Then His fame went throughout all Syria; and they brought to Him all sick people who were afflicted with various diseases and torments, and those who were demon-possessed, epileptics, and paralytics; and He healed them. Great multitudes followed Him—from Galilee, and *from* Decapolis, Jerusalem,

Judea, and beyond the Jordan. And seeing the multitudes, He went up on a mountain, and when He was seated His disciples came to Him. [2] Then He opened His mouth and taught them, saying...'

So basically what we see here is that in the end of Matthew chapter 4, Jesus has gone around, gone around preaching, and teaching and healing people. And for doing this, He has become famous in all Syria, all in Judea, and all the separate surrounding area, and He has become famous for all these wonderful things He is doing. And after this has happened, He doesn't really care that He has all this fame. He just goes up on this mountain, some mountain just to spend some time with his Father, God; so to pray. That's what He's doing up there. And then we find that the disciples come to Jesus because, chapter 6 says Jesus is simply teaching the disciples the ways of life and the ways of truth. The disciples are coming to Jesus wanting to learn from Him and asking Him how to pray.

So I need for you guys to have that sort of attitude, tonight; wanting to come and learn how to pray. Be like the disciples. They realized that there was something real in prayer, so they came to the Lord asking "Teach us to pray."

With those opening statements, Logan explains the power, the necessity, and the results of praying like we should. The final complete content is included when you watch the entire video on the Wikitude app!

Now on to Mark Cahill. He is a powerful speaker and evangelist, who was an Academic all-SEC team member at Auburn University. He attended that Alabama university from 1981 to 1984 on a four-year basketball scholarship and was a teammate of "Sir" Charles Barkley. He earned his bachelor's degree in business.

Shortly after entering the business world, Mark received Jesus Christ as his Savior. This changed his focus, and he began on the road to being an evangelist for the Lord.

Mark Cahill has visited many churches, and he has been to where Logan and I go, the First Baptist Church of Glen Este. It is located in Union Township of Clermont County in the eastern suburbs of Cincinnati, Ohio.

Mark has written several books, framed in logic, common sense, spiritual truth, compassion, creativity, boldness, fearlessness, and woven together with the ideas that anyone can be an active, living, and vibrant example of God's presence.

One powerful book is called: **One Heartbeat Away**

Another one is: **One Thing You Can't Do in Heaven.**

He has written other books and booklets that are so useful, they all should be read.

While speaking at our church, Logan and I had a chance to talk one-on-one with Mark at different times. Mark saw the passion and commitment that Logan had, subsequently blessing him one time with a little spending money.

Logan used the funds wisely and wrote back to Mark explaining how he shared his faith at the restaurant that he went to, and the results that followed. A copy of that letter is shown below. Please read carefully because Logan's muscles were being affected seriously by the disease of Duchenne Muscular Dystrophy and the printing shows the difficulty.

After reading this letter to Mark Cahill from Logan, it makes you think about what happened to the guys mentioned like Gary, Bill, and Steve. If they read this book, will their memory click back to when a young man in a wheelchair shared his faith while dining at that restaurant?

This concludes chapter 21, and there's still more to come!!

Mr. Cahill,

Thank you for taking time to talk to me and sign my book when you came to our church in Cincinnati at First Baptist of Glen Este. My dad and I went out to eat seafood with the generous gift of 50 dollars that you gave me. Thanks again for the money. It was a pretty nice resturaunt, so we actually had three waitors serving us. Of course we eventually witnessed to all three of them. The first one, Gary, quickly and boldly told us he was a born again Christian. Next was Bill, who grew up in a Christian home and was saved, but he had some questions about his faith. Steve was lost and he was looking for answers. We got their addresses and are sending them books. I am trying to share my faith at school. Thank you for inspiring me!

Sincerely, Logan Shannon

Chapter 22

Logan's Letter to God

Dear God,

To be honest, it feels a little weird to write this letter because I have such easy access to You with prayer. And You know as well as I do (actually better), just how much I need the outlet of prayer to continually converse with You. I do my best to access it as much as possible, and there is no doubt that it's one of my, if not my most, favorite things to do! I love You, Lord, and want to give You all of me because you're worthy of that and so much more! You know that some of my greatest prayers are to be a man after your own heart like David, to have your wisdom poured over me like Solomon, and to have my words never fall to the ground like Samuel. But, more than anything, I just want to be known by You and to know You more.

My desire is to be closer to you each day. I hope my heart is pure and true to that desire in Your eyes; and if it is not, make me a clean vessel for Your service! Mold me and make me after Your will and always adjust mine to match Yours.

Heavenly Father, You also know I am continually praying **and** believing for a manifestation of physical healing from Duchenne Muscular Dystrophy (DMD). Honestly, I don't need to be healed in order to follow You, but I just **know** that is in Your plan for me and everyone else! If it doesn't manifest itself in this life, we can know perfection is in store for us in Heaven! I rely on You alone in this area because I know You are the only one who offers any true hope in the circumstance. Strengthen me as You use the trial and the triumph to make an impact for Your kingdom!

I also rely completely on You in my desire for a romantic relationship. As with the previous situation, You know my heart is that I don't need this in order to follow You. But, (though this seems less severe to probably everyone looking on from outside) You know from my prayers, and the unique personality You've given me, that the romantic relationship situation is just as hard for me to face as DMD. I will continue to call out with all my heart for You to comfort and guide me through these circumstances.

I also lift up everyone I know, and do not know, that is going through some sort of trial, whether it be health issues like I've faced, relational issues or unfulfilled desires, financial lack, or dreams that have not been met. Sometimes I'm going through so much that I won't pray as much for others as I should and I'm sure they can relate with that. Unify the body of Christ and lift our heads up as we lift each other up to You!

I'm sure many people are holding on to the Scripture, John 14:14, which says, "Ask ANYTHING in my name, and I will do it." I believe that You mean just what You say in that statement. But help others (and even me), to better understand that this means we'll receive it in Your timing and according to the will You have set up for our lives. I know many expect for that to mean that as soon as they ask for something from You, it will be given to them, because I definitely went through a period where I thought this way.

We think we'll get completely fixed up in a short period of time following our prayer, but more often than not it happens over a long period with many painful bumps and lessons along the way.

That's the way life is designed in its current fallen nature. I've been through it and You've revealed to me that there's no automatic simple answer to life's difficult questions. We simply do not know the fullness of Your perfect plan. Deep faith and complete trust in You is what we must keep our focus on; You are the hope we cling to! Again, strengthen and be with me and the rest of Your created people. Thank you for the extent of Your love for me! Thank You for creating me and maintaining my life! Thank You that You will never leave me or forsake me! I love You and choose to always follow You, Lord!

Your Beloved Child,
Logan

Chapter 23

Why Baptism?

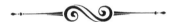

T here is an element of uniqueness in a Christian relationship between a person and God where a dramatic symbol takes place, and that's baptism. Pastor Brent Snook had the privilege of baptizing Logan after his profession in his faith that Jesus Christ is the Son of God who was sent to be the redeemer of humanity.

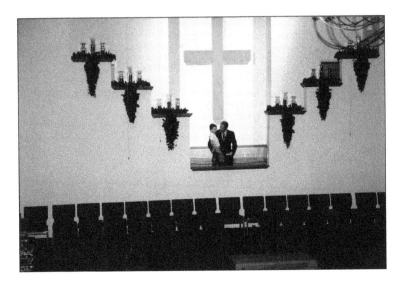

Almost all baptisms at our church proceed by the new believer walking down into a tank of water called the baptismal. It could be a river, pool, or other available water source, but the in-church facility provides a clean and convenient alternative. Logan knew he would follow Christ's example of baptism, and due to the progressive weakness developing in his muscles, Pastor Snook held Logan and baptized him.

There are many places where "baptism" is mentioned in God's Word. So, what exactly is that? What does the Bible mean when it says "baptize" or "baptism"? There are root words and many forms in the Greek language, but all point to a submersion or "burial" of some sort. The studies on this word are exhaustive, and this chapter touches on the simplest of explanations without getting into the tall grass of every possible interpretation.

Acts chapter 2, verse 38 says – "Then Peter said to them, 'Repent, and let every one of you be baptized in the name of Jesus Christ for the remission of sins; and you shall receive the gift of the Holy Spirit.' " It says repent (first) and then be baptized (second) in that order. It means a person must willingly and physically understand "repent" before the action of baptism. Logan Shannon received the Holy Spirit through Jesus Christ into his heart at a young age, and was baptized to show evidence of this decision in his life. The picture above shows Logan being put 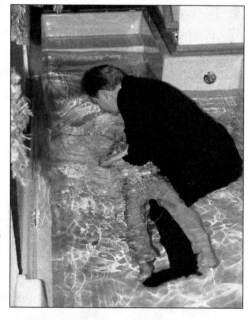 under the surface of the water, almost in a horizontal position.

So what exactly happened to Logan? What came over him to see a need to take action in his spiritual life? Let's start by a quick study on how mankind has the mindset to reject God's ways. Every person was born with sinful ways but hasn't admitted they are sinful and in need of a Redeemer. God reveals to each person the right way to His heart and His heaven, and they choose whether to receive Him or reject Him. Logan decided to accept Him! Even as Logan's limbs were beginning to fail, he still wanted to obey his God, his Savior, Jesus Christ, and the Holy Spirit by being baptized.

Repentance means turning away from a sinful, self-centered way of life apart from the way that God wants us to live. Self-imposed lifestyle corrections without God are not permanent, and falling back into previous destructive habits is commonplace. A

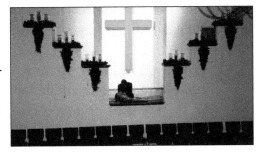

permanent turning away comes from the acceptance of redemption from sinful behavior through the substitutionary death of Jesus Christ. He paid the highest possible price for us by being the **perfect** one and **only** one that could do it.

So fully trusting in what He did to make our sin payment allows the "original person" or "old man" to be transformed into a new person. That redemption comes by each person individually inviting the Spirit of God through Jesus Christ to take over their life. It is the voluntary submission to a Holy God that transitions us from "old man" to "new man". So how does anyone know this really happened? How does family, how do friends, how does anyone know that a change really took place? There HAS to be some outward expression, or visual evidence, and Jesus made **baptism** that action to show physically and visibly what happened internally and invisibly.

So, the transitional death of the "old man" by being put "under" (like the dirt in a burial) continues by revealing the "new man" who emerges from the grave as a raised and genuinely new person with a new set of behaviors.

If we are to "bury" that old man (horizontal position), we should dig a hole in the ground, cover the person up for a proper burial, and dig them back out for a proper raising to begin walking in their new life. But, boy that's inconvenient, dangerous, and really messy and time consuming! The Lord used water for that outward and visual picture of a death (going under), and raising to walk in newness of life (coming back up) for efficiency, vividness, and identification. Look at the picture on the previous page to see Logan being brought back out of the water.

We can visually see that it's the same person (no name change or fingerprint alterations), but what happened INSIDE is what made the "new" person. That regenerative spiritual cleansing internally is what can't be seen except by a changed lifestyle.

> Romans chapter 6, verse 6 – "...knowing this, that our **old man** was crucified with *Him,* that the body of sin might be done away with, that we should no longer be slaves of sin."

> Ephesians chapter 4, verse 22 – "...that you put off, concerning your former conduct, the **old man** which grows corrupt according to the deceitful lusts..."

> Colossians chapter 3, verse 9 – "Do not lie to one another, since you have put off the **old man** with his deeds..."

So, what does the original language of the New Testament say about "baptize" and "baptism"? The original Greek root word for "baptize"(English): βαπτίζω, pronounced "baptidzo".

> Romans Chapter 6, verses 1–4: "[1] What shall we say then? Shall we continue in sin that grace may abound? [2] Certainly not! How shall we who died to sin live any longer in it? [3] Or do you not know that as many of us as were **baptized** into Christ Jesus

were **baptized** into His death? [4] Therefore we were buried with Him through baptism into death, that just as Christ was raised from the dead by the glory of the Father, even so we also should walk in newness of life."

From the first part of verse 3: ὅτι ὅσοι **ἐβαπτίσθημεν** εἰς Χριστὸν means "...those who have been **baptized** into Christ".

From the last part of verse 3: θάνατον αὐτοῦ **ἐβαπτίσθημεν** means "...have been **baptized** into His death."

So the picture is death and raising back up. Why was this vividly important, and why were followers of Jesus Christ commanded to do this? In many places the Bible quotes "putting off the old man."

Galatians 3:27 – "For as many of you as were baptized into Christ have put on Christ."

εἰς Χριστὸν **ἐβαπτίσθητε** Χριστὸν ἐνεδύσασθε means "...those who were baptized into Christ..."

Colossians chapter 2, verse 12: "....buried with Him in **baptism**, in which you also were raised with *Him* through faith in the working of God, who raised Him from the dead."

So, these pictures show evidence that Logan followed the instructions of "repent and be baptized".

A Closing Word From Logan

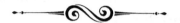

Dear Readers,

As we come to the end of this creative look at the journey of my life thus far, I would like to give you a few overall encompassing thoughts that I have regarding both broadly my life as a whole, and this specific piece of writing meant to get my life's message out.

Let me begin by sharing this: This life is certainly not one that I wanted or

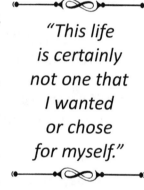

"This life is certainly not one that I wanted or chose for myself."

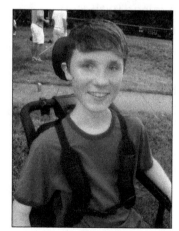

chose for myself. Truthfully, if it were up to me, I would have come into this world just like everyone else, without any of the diverse effects of Duchenne Muscular Dystrophy. And if it were up to me now, God's healing hand would deliver me completely from the condition with the snap of His finger. That's because in many ways I feel as though every possible purpose for the situation has been fulfilled (which of course, is not up to me). But these are feelings we all have when it comes to life's difficulties.

To put it more simply, this isn't easy! This isn't enjoyable! This isn't clear at all! But I have and will always continue pushing forward as I hold on to the hope and promise of brighter days that are sure to come in the future!

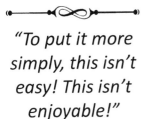

"To put it more simply, this isn't easy! This isn't enjoyable!"

And as hard as it all can be, I'm generally okay with that since I am able to take hold of the Creator of everything we see, as He is taking hold of me, never to let go!

Yes, I'm telling you once again, as I'm sure you've become accustomed to by now, the theme that I point everything back to, that anything positive that comes from my struggles, including my outlook on it all, is due only to my Lord, Jesus, and the rela-

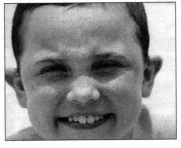

tionship He has graciously enabled me to have with Him! That is the gift I have been given; that is the gift I have been sent to share with you.

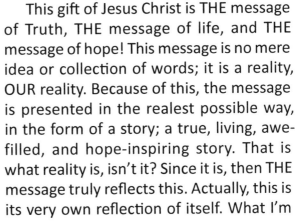

"My life's story is only a minute fraction of THE story, but it is still a story that needed to be told, just as every single story must be told."

This gift of Jesus Christ is THE message of Truth, THE message of life, and THE message of hope! This message is no mere idea or collection of words; it is a reality, OUR reality. Because of this, the message is presented in the realest possible way, in the form of a story; a true, living, awe-filled, and hope-inspiring story. That is what reality is, isn't it? Since it is, then THE message truly reflects this. Actually, this is its very own reflection of itself. What I'm telling you is that this message, THE message, is THE story of EVERYTHING. It IS reality.

The interesting dynamic of THE message or story, is that it contains story upon story upon story within itself. In fact, every true story that has ever existed is a part of THE story! Though not every story, as most of the stories in our reality are about men with free will, chooses to fall in line with THE message (which is the overarching plan and purpose of all things). The Storyteller still works all into the telling of THE story. Each story, or perhaps the main character of each story, can either make a decision to join in with THE main character, who is The Storyteller of THE story, or reject His storyboard for his own. That choice is what every story rests upon.

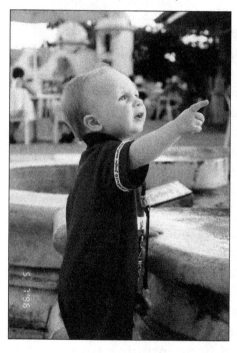

My life's story is only a minute fraction of THE story, but it is still a story that needed to be told, just as every single story must be told. And as the character of my story, I chose long ago to join in with the One in charge of all things and willingly allow His way to be done, in order for THE message to be spread.

That is why I do what I do, say what I say, and live how I live. Of course, as I have recounted to you before, I am not necessarily a fan of the course of events my story has entailed. Even with this being true, in the deepest sense humanly possible I understand the purpose and benefits of the seemingly endless series of valleys within one major valley that is woven into the story of my life. It has produced great levels of wisdom, maturity, and perseverance in faith within me that I know would never have grown or become evident outside of the battle. I am able to say this, not to boast, but simply because it is true. That is the nature of THE message; a nature of conquering evil with grace; a nature of overcoming death with redemption! It brings forth hope out of every hurt! It takes grief and turns it into good! From every great trial it creates an even greater triumph!

"There will be questions to come that you must ask, and every one of those questions has a sufficient answer. I know this because I have wrestled with God with plenty of my own questions; and without fail, He has always provided me with some sort of explanation."

This has been true for me, and it can be true for you! In fact, it will ultimately be true for all those who choose to believe. That's the condition, you <u>must</u> believe!

There is enough evidence and proof based on what I've told you (and beyond) in order to realize the validity of the entirety of this Truth I send to you, through whom I have been sent, for one to make their decision. The choice is entirely yours, no pressure from or on anyone else; but perhaps some pressure within yourself. Whether you find it all accurate or not, the rest of your life can, and very well will, hinge on this very decision. ***Every experience has endless impact***. This is all consistent with the reality we see and face each day.

There will be questions to come that you must ask, and every one of those questions has a sufficient answer. I know this because I have wrestled with God with plenty of my own questions, and without fail, He has always provided me with some sort of explanation.

You are not alone in any of this so there is nothing to fear, but it is important to clearly consider and examine what has been presented as you arrive at a place of choosing. But my words alone are not a deep or strong enough foundation for you to base your choice upon; therefore, I must share with you what the Lord of everything Himself says about the matter, which is, really, the core matter of all life.

So, in the spirit of letters, let's bring everything home and to a close, by looking directly into God's own personal letter to us, His Word, The Bible. In this letter that God has written to us, He has given us all that we need to understand the purposes of virtually everything, and even laid out for us how to live life as effectively as possible. Seriously, you name it and the Bible has something to say about it. Everything that is in the God-breathed Letter meant for us, points to the most important aspect of Truth found in its pages: the means of attaining and sustaining a reconciled relationship with our Heavenly Father. This is His heart and deepest desire, to have an intimate, alive relationship with His created children. To obtain this reconciliation, through the way He has provided, translates to an eternal, perfect fellowship with Him.

"So, in the spirit of letters, let's bring everything home and to a close by looking directly into God's own personal letter to us, His Word, the Bible."

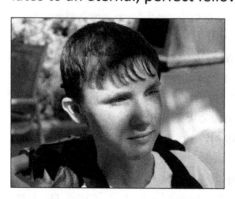

Now you can see why reconciling us to Him is so important to God. It is the focal point of THE story that He has put in motion and Word He has divinely written. He wants to be with us and us to be with Him. Out of His great love for all of us, He provided the manner to accomplish just that and further, has presented it to us in a clear, fully preserved form. So, here are a few of the highlights of this final reconciliation in His letter...

To start with, here's a verse that sums up His entire plan of restoring our relationship with Him, found in John 3:16, "For God so loved the world that He gave His only begotten Son, that whoever believes in Him should not perish but have everlasting life."

And that only begotten Son of His, that was sent for us, was, and is, Jesus Christ Himself. And as I've said before, all that is required of each of us is a simple belief that Jesus is the sent Savior for us to be reconciled with God. I believe, and this IS the foundation of my entire life.

But let me break down all that the verse entails through explanation provided in other passages. In Romans 3:10 we read, "As it is written: 'There is none righteous, no, not one.'" None of us are righteous (good from the perfection standpoint) in comparison to God's standard, because each of us has gone after our own ways instead of His in some manner.

We have all **traded the Truth** for some sort of lie that is pleasing to our minds. Later on in Romans 3:23, it says, "For all have sinned and fall short of the glory of God." Because of the sin (or lack of righteousness) that we have committed, we fall astronomically short of the perfect goodness of God.

With this being the case, we cannot realistically survive in His presence, let alone have a personal relationship with a Holy God. Thankfully, we find Jesus' sacrificial provision for our redemption again in

"Out of His great love for all of us, He provided the manner to accomplish just that; and further, has presented it to us in a clear, fully preserved form."

"But God demonstrates His own love for us, in that while we were still sinners, Christ died for us. Romans 5:8."

Romans 5:8, "But God demonstrates His own love toward us, in that while we were still sinners, Christ died for us." You see, God loved us in our filthy disobedience to the extent that He was able to look past our shortcomings. He gave us Jesus to be righteousness imputed on our behalf, and the sacrifice that was made for

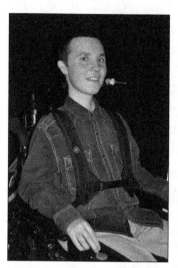

us was Jesus' very life and shed blood.

Much to the same effect, but with a little more weight, in Romans 6:23 it is written, "For the wages of sin is death, but the gift of God is eternal life in Christ Jesus our Lord." Our sins are so dirty in comparison to God's perfection, that the penalty we are owed for them is both physical death and spiritual death, resulting in eternal separation from God. But again, that is not what God wants for us. He gifted us with the life, sacrificial crucifixion, and resurrection of Christ, from the dead, to enable our restored relationship with Him. This love and grace of the Father is beautiful beyond compare, and time and time again the Lord has proven the Truth of THIS good news in the details of my life. He desires to do the same in yours!

To solidify the Truth of the Gospel of Christ, as I have just presented it to you, here are the words of Isaiah. He was a prophet that predicted the sacrifice of Jesus for our salvation centuries before it even occurred in the book of Isaiah, chapter 53:5-6, "But He was wounded for our transgressions, He was bruised for our iniquities; the chastisement for our peace was upon Him, and by His stripes we are healed. All we like sheep

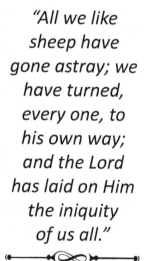

"All we like sheep have gone astray; we have turned, every one, to his own way; and the Lord has laid on Him the iniquity of us all."

have gone astray; we have turned, every one, to his own way; and the Lord has laid on Him the iniquity of us all."

Here is described exactly what Jesus went through for our sake; being beaten, bruised, and crucified for our pursuit of sin. He bore our punishment so that we could wear His perfect righteousness, and upon the reception and belief of Christ as Savior, all of His followers are rewarded with the many promises of His salvation.

In fact, in the end of all things, when eternity is reached, we are also told in Isaiah 25:8 that, "He will swallow up death forever, and the Lord God will wipe away tears from all faces; the rebuke of His people He will take away from all the earth; for the Lord has spoken." The story that God wills and desires for all of us who are undeserving of His grace and goodness is the most amazing and fulfilling thing you can ever take part in! I have found this to be none less than 100% true, and Jesus Christ has impacted my life with the call and ability to hopefully impact many more lives for Him!

Because "He personally bore our sins in His [own] body on the tree {as on an altar and offered Himself on it}, that we might die to sin and live to righteousness.", as 1 Peter 2:24 (AMP) says, anyone and everyone can come to Jesus and receive Him as their personal Lord and Savior! God literally, by his grace, did all the work for us; all anyone has to do is receive the gift! A simple call out to the Father, in con-

"...anyone and everyone can come to Jesus and receive Him as their Lord and Savior!"

fessing your sins and turning away from them, then asking (out of belief that He is the Son of God) that Jesus, the Author of Salvation, would be their reconciled Lord, is all that is required to claim His saving peace. To make the point, He declares in Acts 2:21 (AMP), "And it shall be that whoever shall call upon the name of the Lord [invoking, adoring, and worshiping the Lord – Christ] shall be saved."

So, there you have it – To believe in Christ, and call on His perfect name, is alone enough to save your soul and renew your spirit. Invoke His shed blood to receive forgiveness, adore Him for His extended righteousness, and worship Him as director of your life. You will not become immediately perfect (thankfully God doesn't even expect this), but in the resurrection of your spiritual life through Him, you will receive such unprecedented joy, peace, and purpose, that your life will never be the same!

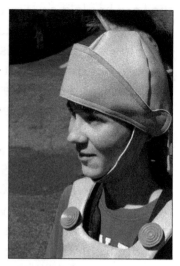

I can promise all this to be true for you because it is so very true of what He has done for me and what He has done for Lee! Don't let His gift for your life pass you by for even a moment; there's no time to waste!

Finally, let's look at Romans 8:38-39 (AMP) to see the assurance of Christ's permanent salvation for those who follow Him: "For I am persuaded beyond doubt (am sure) that neither death nor life, nor angels nor principalities, nor things impending and threatening, nor things to come, nor powers, nor height, nor depth, nor anything else in all creation will be able to separate us from the love of God which is in Christ Jesus our Lord." There is absolutely nothing that could ever pluck us from God's hand and remove the all-covering love of Christ! Every blessing that Jesus gives can never be taken away, every storm that is endured will be used for our good, and everything that we do can be done for

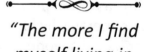

"The more I find myself living in Christ, the more of my true self I find. I mean this with all that is within me!"

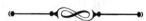

His glory! That is what I have chosen to believe and live by, and I pray that you may do the same!

Before I let you close this book and store its pages away, I have one more thing to say: To echo the heartbeat of something that C. S. Lewis once wrote, in my own words; The more I find myself living in Christ, the more of my true self I find. I mean this with all that is within me! This is exactly what Jesus meant for us. After all, we were created for Him in the first place. It is my hope, that from reading my story, and observing my life, you would be challenged to at least examine whether the gospel of Christ, the foundation of my life as you have read, is the truth or not; and attempt, through His grace, to experience the abundant life that He has provided for me, my family, and many of my friends. Thanks for coming along with us to intimately encounter the richness of my life through letters and the rest! Let it impact you to impact the lives of others. I look forward to connecting with or meeting with each one of you, in accordance to God's will!

You can reach me on social media in the following ways: Twitter & Instagram – @TheLoganShannon and on Facebook - Logan Shannon Page.

God Bless You All,
Logan Shannon

Luke 5:18-24 says:

Then behold, men brought on a bed a man who was paralyzed, whom they sought to bring in and lay before Him. And
when they could not find how they might bring him in, because
of the crowd, they went up on the housetop and let him down
with *his* bed through the tiling into the midst before Jesus.

When He saw their faith, He said to him, "Man, your sins are
forgiven you." And the scribes and the Pharisees began to reason,
saying, "Who is this who speaks blasphemies? Who can forgive
sins but God alone?"

But when Jesus perceived their thoughts, He answered and
said to them, "Why are you reasoning in your hearts? Which is
easier, to say, 'Your sins are forgiven you,' or to say, 'Rise up and
walk'? But that you may know that the Son of Man has power on
earth to forgive sins"—He said to the man who was paralyzed, "I
say to you, arise, take up your bed, and go to your house."

Psalm 30:2-5 says:

O LORD my God, I cried out to You, and You healed me.
O LORD, You brought my soul up from the grave;
You have kept me alive, that I should not go down to the pit.
Sing praise to the LORD, you saints of His,
And give thanks at the remembrance of His holy name.
For His anger *is but for* a moment, His favor *is for* life;
Weeping may endure for a night, But joy *comes* in the morning.

The Future...

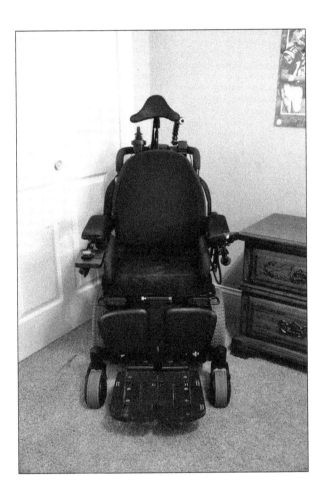

Epilogue

L ogan knows that the world won't stop after this book. Things will never stay the same. So where do you, the reader fit in now? Where is the impact that you will make on others with your life? Look back and recall how you've lived, and what impressions have been made, or lives have been changed through your influence. Imagine how writing a letter of your own to someone who really made a difference will affect their lives as well.

Logan will continue to be part of people's lives; and will offer sound counsel, humorous anecdotes, and plenty of encouragement. Some may have felt that wonderful touch from someone who has shared a heart-felt letter and brought them a slice of joy and happiness.

But, above all, Logan wants every reader to experience the peace that comes with trusting Jesus Christ with their lives. Logan knows there are temptations at every corner; he knows the pressure that we can be under, yet, he experiences his life completely dependent on others for daily living. He wants each one of you to trust God the same way. He is praying you will!

After all, as Logan said, God wrote a special "letter" to everyone called the Holy Bible. It is to be used for everyone's benefit, and for receiving a glorious crown to be worn in heaven. You need to respond to God's letter by receiving Jesus Christ as your personal Savior for the remission of your sins, and walk in the newness of life. Logan and I have! The benefits are out of this world!

Credits

We want to thank everyone who contributed to this effort through writing letters, reviews, and offering insight. The Shannon family knows the significance of time that was invested from all who submitted letters and pictures. Logan's experiences with the large circle of friends revealed the impact that one life can make.

Our deepest thanks to our entire publishing team at Xulon Press, especially Michael Caryl who was our original contact, and our project coordinator, Jennifer Kasper, for your interest in the project and all of the hard work and patience that went into the publication of The Logan Letters! We couldn't have done it without you!"

Thank you to our copy proofreader and being the "eyes of the editor", Mrs. Paula Goodnight of Murfreesboro, Tennessee. She is known for exemplary work, and we appreciate the high standard that was maintained throughout. Her first phase reviews provided vital revisions for clarification and understanding.

writenow.paula@gmail.com is how to contact her.

Thank you to Stephanie Trammell for all the final editing and reviews once the book sections were complete. You have added positive counsel and recommendations, bringing improvements to the overall readability of this book.

Contact: stephanie34@zoomtown.com

Thank you to Eric Anthony Cieslewicz, producer for the EntreLeadership podcast. You went over and above our expectations with your review process. Your content editing expertise and input was invaluable.

https://www.entreleadership.com

Thank you to Mr. Stacy Doose of Cincinnati, Ohio, for all the video talent he brought to the table. His interviews were relaxed and heart-felt. Historical excellence prevailed, and readers are able to "see" how Logan made impressions. Stacy is a first-class individual and can be contacted:

stacy@chilidogpictures.com

Thank you to Dale Stoops of One Stop Print Solutions for guidance and pertinent printing and construction information. His experience provided valuable insight into publishing and other media features. Contact Dale at:

www.onestopprintsolutions.com

Thank you to David Braughler of Braughler Books. He has many years of printing experience and shared important aspects for this project. Contact Dave at:

https://braughlerbooks.com

Thank you to Gina Gundersen and Jennifer Craig of Daubenmire's Printing, Middletown, Ohio for the graphic design of the cover and the organization of the picture sections. Their experience and talent provided value and visual interest to the content of the book. Contact them at:

www.daubenmiresprinting.com.

Thank you to Brant Hansen, an American radio personality who has hosted the morning show on the national Christian radio WAY-FM Network and the afternoon show on the national Christian radio network Air1, and author of the book, "Unoffendable: How Just One Change Can Make All of Life Better." Brant has offered positive comments about this book.

www.branthansen.com

Thank you Julie Simpson, and Larry and Paula Bussard for your photographic skills and contributions. You have added tremendous value and imagery to the special look of this work. Thank you, Tyra Shannon, for searching through hundreds of older and current photographs, for the right mix from which final selections could be made.

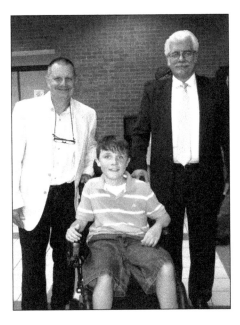

Steve Brungs was an 8th grade teacher at the Glen Este Middle School. When Logan was in his class, a special project on history was assigned and Logan chose me to help him regarding things that happened in the 1960's. It was that combined effort several years ago that may have birthed us working together. The picture shown is Logan in 8th grade, his teacher, Steve Brungs, and me posing at the conclusion to the project.

CPSIA information can be obtained
at www.ICGtesting.com
Printed in the USA
BVHW012151260919
559594BV00004B/56/P